LET'S
GET
NAKE

501 RIDICULOUSLY HOT Sex Mo

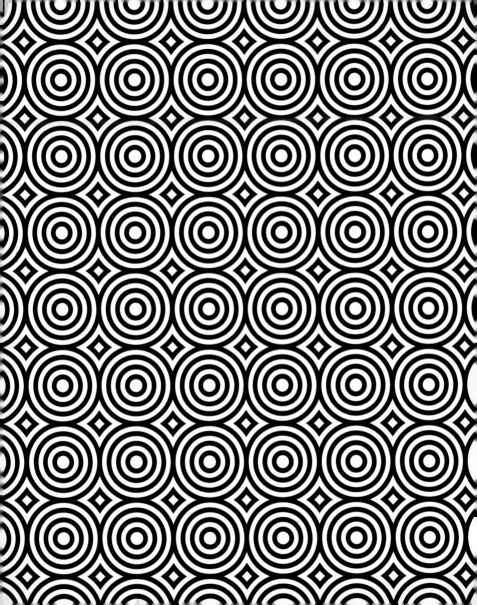

COSMO's

LET'S

GET

NAKED

501 RIDICULOUSLY HOT Sex Moves

From the editors of COSMOPOLITAN

HEARST BOOKS
New York

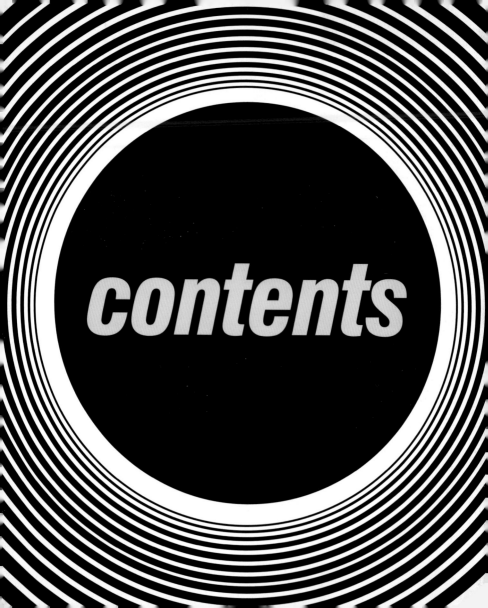

contents

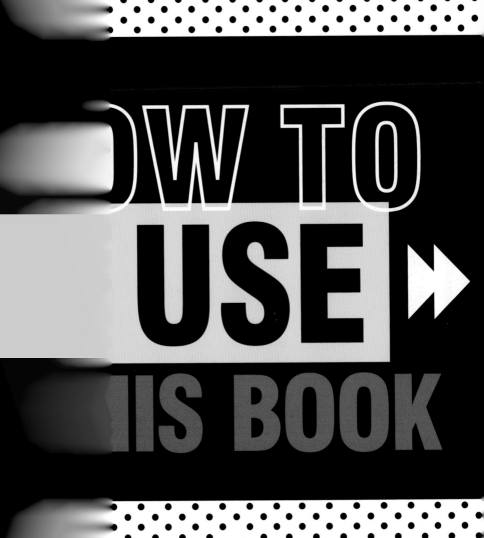

OW TO
USE ▶▶
IS BOOK

ALL SKILLS TAKE
PRACTICE.

Cooking. Violin. Achieving the perfect salon blowout on your own. **Sex is no different:** Anyone can *do* it, but if you want to have the best sex ever, you've got to hit the books *and* the sheets.

So let this book be your textbook for the art of ridiculously hot sex. We'll start out with the basics and work our way up to the advanced tips and tricks for the most bangin' sex life ever. (Pun intended, obvs.)

the warm-up

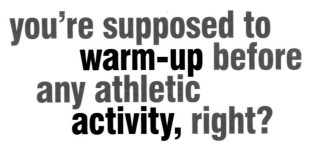

you're supposed to warm-up before any athletic activity, right?

Sex, obviously, is no different, but when it comes to having truly amazing, **next-level sex**, sometimes it's your mind that needs to get into the game as well as your body. In this section of the book, we're gonna map out some warm-up **exercises**, from solo sex to sexting, to get you in tune with your sexiest self and primed for the **best sex** of your life. . . .

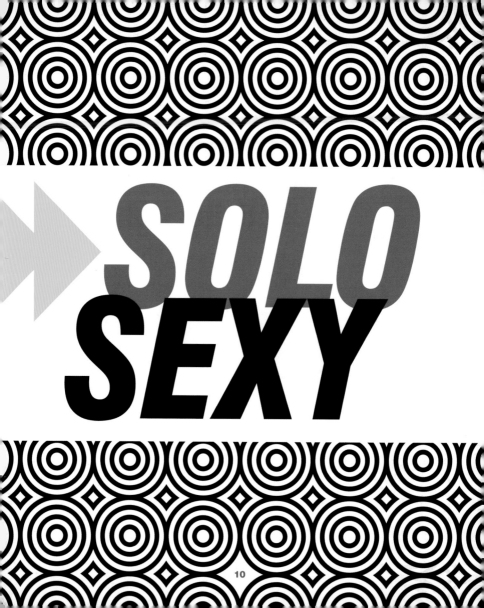

SOLO
SEXY

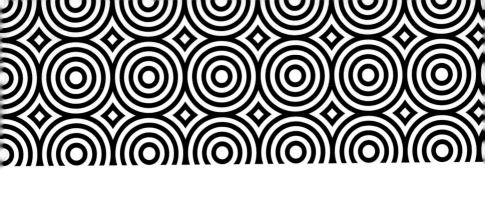

Whether you're **PLEASING YOURSELF** or teaching your guy how to work your love button, the first step toward a **SATISFYING SEX LIFE** is getting to know your own turn-ons so you can reach your **HIGH NOTE** any time.

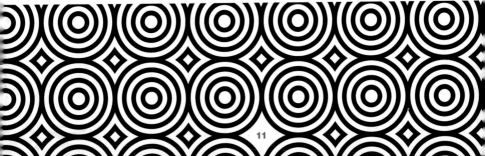

GET into
an *orgasmic*
state
of MIND

LADYGASMS are composed of
the right mind-set and the right moves.
These mental and physical tips
(and a little practice) will help you
find your happy place.

1 READ OR WATCH SOME SEXY STUFF.
Whether you're turned on by erotica, porn, or a hot indie band, partake in that activity before engaging in sexy-time.

2 HAVE A GLASS OF WINE.
Not only will it help you de-stress, it'll increase circulation and blood flow to your pelvis, which is necessary to orgasm.

3 ELIMINATE DISTRACTIONS.
It's hard to get off when you're thinking about work/your to-do list/the pile of laundry that you've been meaning to put away for three days now, etc. Turn off your phone, light candles, take a bath—whatever will help you get in the mood, and out of your own head.

4 START WITH MANUAL.
Rather than going straight for the vibrator, start slow with manual stimulation, applying light pressure to your clitoris and labia. (Adding a water-based lube will enhance your pleasure.)

5 DON'T FREAK OUT IF IT DOESN'T FEEL LIKE IT'LL HAPPEN.
On average, it takes a woman 20 minutes of direct stimulation to have an orgasm (some women take more or less—and that's normal as well). It's common to reach a plateau phase, when you're turned on but feel like you've stalled. Don't lose hope. Stick with what got you to that point and you'll likely get there. If not, you probably will next time!

SOME SEXY SUGGESTIONS

Books: *Fifty Shades of Grey*, by E. L. James; *Delta of Venus*, by Anaïs Nin; *Fanny Hill*, by John Cleland

Movies: *I Am Love*, *Savages*, *Atonement*, *The Notebook*

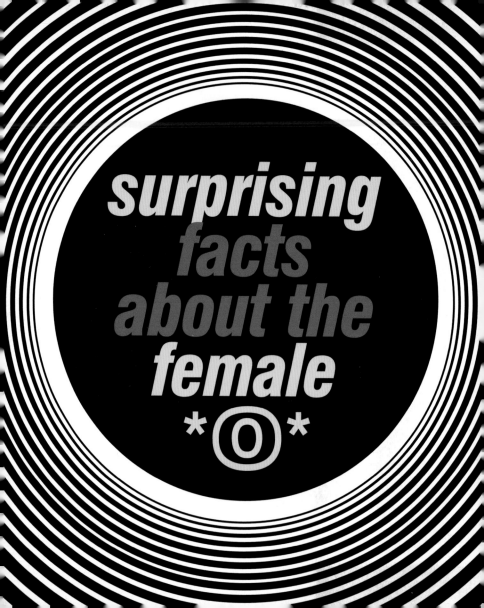

1 You're **more likely** to orgasm if your feet are **warm...** (Another reason to surprise him in thigh-highs!)

2 The typical female **orgasm** lasts **twenty-five seconds.**

3 A woman's odds of **climaxing** increase as she **ages.**

4 Women can have **wet dreams.** They usually happens during the **REM** sleep cycle, when blood flow to the vagina increases.

5 Fourteen percent of women have experienced a so-called **zone orgasm**, which happens when a part of the body other than the **boobs**, clitoris, or vagina is stimulated.

6 In a recent Indiana University study, 51 percent of women reported having an O during an **abdominal exercise . . .** and it's not just crunches. Nearly 30 percent of women said they experienced an orgasm while weight lifting, and **20 percent** did while practicing yoga.

SOLO SEX MOVES ▶▶

Sexy ways to get down with your bad girl self.

BEGINNING

fancy
fingers

Fingers are the **perfect tools** for learning which sensations, speeds, and rhythms can get you off. Get playful and draw the alphabet with your pinkie. Or try lightly tapping your clitoris with one finger, **speeding up** as you become aroused. All the while, note areas and touches that provide the most satisfaction. It takes trial and error to figure out what makes you tick. **Experiment**, and you'll be surprised by the sexy sensations you can provoke.

INTERMEDIATE

the figure eight

Use one or more fingers to **glide up,** over, and around your clitoral area, tracing the number eight. You'll cover the clitoris and the inner labia—a **lusty locale** that has nerve endings within its walls, which some women find even **more arousing** than the clitoris.

ADVANCED

the three-fingers thrill

Use your index and ring fingers to **hold open** your labia. This frees up your middle finger to **stroke** the tip of your clitoris.

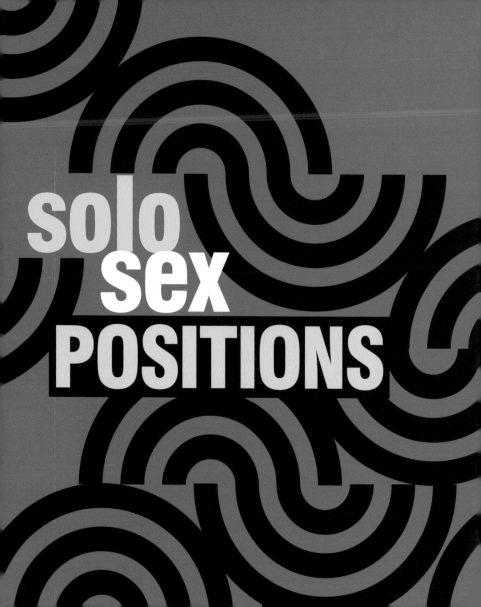

THE FUMBLING STRANGER

You feel like trying **something new** tonight, so use your opposite hand to masturbate. It'll feel weird, almost like you're **fooling around** with someone for the first time, and that's what makes it so **completely hot**.

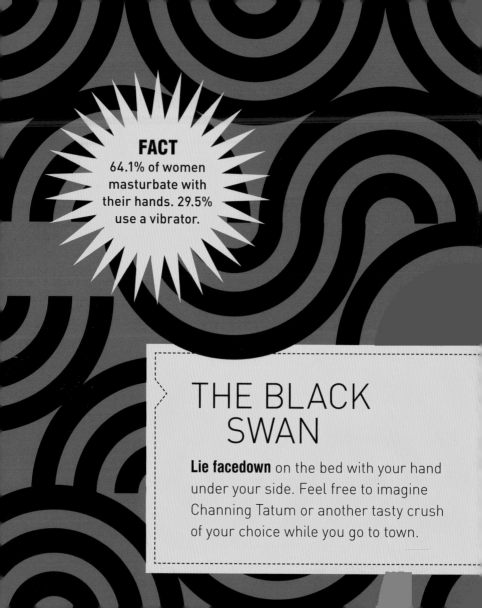

FACT

64.1% of women masturbate with their hands. 29.5% use a vibrator.

THE BLACK SWAN

Lie facedown on the bed with your hand under your side. Feel free to imagine Channing Tatum or another tasty crush of your choice while you go to town.

THE LONG
WAY AROUND

Missionary gets boring even with
solo sex, so **lie facedown** on a pillow,
take your hand, and put it behind you,
coming between your legs. Use the
pillow to **muffle your moans.**

I *masturbate* a lot. Like, every day. Is there any *medical* *reason* why it's bad for me?

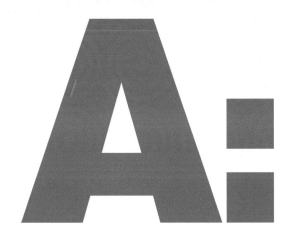

As long as you're not so obsessed with masturbating that you're missing work to lock yourself in your room, blast the Divinyls' "I Touch Myself," and get down with a feather tickler you've affectionately named Tim Riggins, then no. Touching yourself is actually good for your health. It relieves tension and releases the flow of the same endorphins that flow post-workout. Think of it as a hookup with someone fantastic: you!

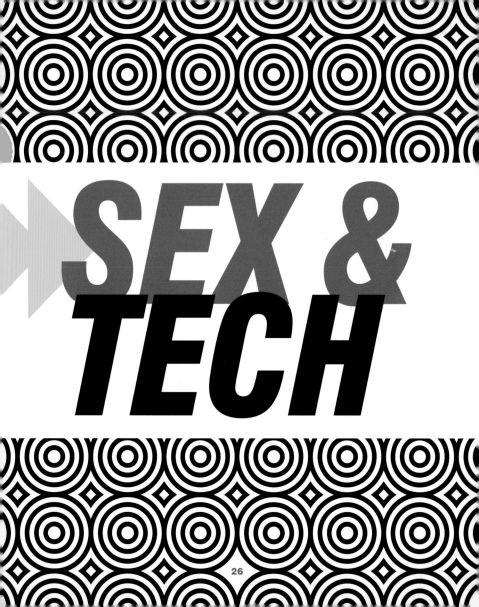

SEX & TECH

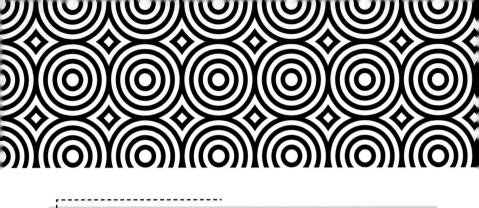

These days, your most **VERSATILE** sex toy is your phone: convenient, **MULTIFACETED**, and, let's face it, always with you. In this section, we'll show you how to use it to **REV UP** your engine—without ending up as the lead story on TMZ . . .

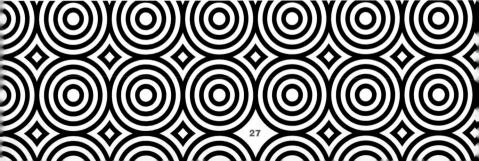

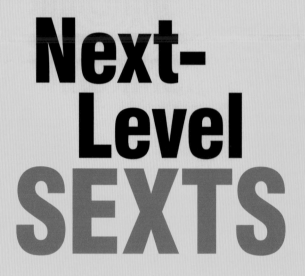

Next-Level SEXTS

The best SEXTS are like great foreplay—they're spicy but still leave a little to the imagination. Find out how to max out your sext appeal here.

~~TONGUE~~ FINGER-TIED? TRY OUT THESE SAMPLE SEXTS:

1 "I've been daydreaming about you all day at work. I can't concentrate thinking about what I'm going to do to you when I get home."

2 "Sitting at my desk fantasizing about how hot it would be to do it in my office."

3 "I can't stop thinking about last night. Are you as ready for round two as I am?"

SHOW YOUR SEXT-Y SIDE ▶▶

PRO TIP: A smiley face masquerading as an O-face is never not funny.

CORRUPT YOUR FAVORITE EMOJI—and your boyfriend's mind—all without saying a single word. Graduate from a standard-issue sext to a sextmoji, a genius string of emoji used to inspire boners.

    suggests post-work shower sex.

    Someone's getting a retro handjob!

SEND A NAUGHTY PUZZLE Introduce him to the saucy slideshow sext. Start snapping selfies of your hot-ass self from the floor up—ankles, calves—and then start over from the shoulders down: Think collarbone, décolletage. Just when he thinks some money shots are coming his way, tell him he has a road map for his mouth to follow tonight.

SEXTING SEXTING 123 Tap into the Voice Memos app on your smartphone and tell him what you want to do to him later. Send it in a text message—he'll be pleasantly surprised to hear your naughty voice purring dirty, dirty things.

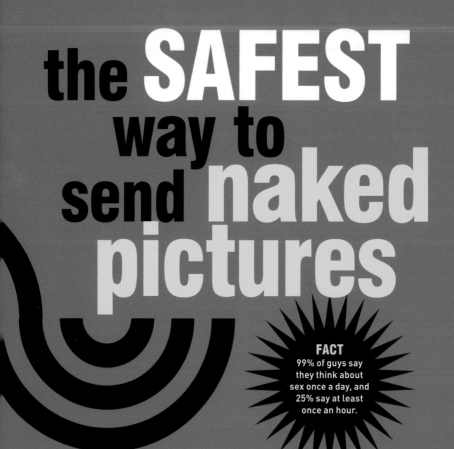

the SAFEST way to send naked pictures

FACT
99% of guys say they think about sex once a day, and 25% say at least once an hour.

THE GOLDEN RULE OF NAKED PICS is that there's absolutely nothing wrong with taking **naked pics,** whether it's a turn-on for you or your BF (or both). But there is something *very* wrong with people who leak nude photos that were intended for their eyes only and with hackers who steal nude photos from the Cloud. Do you trust your boyfriend is a stand-up guy who won't share your **saucy snaps,** but you're worried about your pics winding up in the hands of some evil hacker? Tech experts recommend downloading an app like Threema or KeepSafe. They hide your pics behind a password that you can share with your BF so that once you send your saucy in-the-mirror butt selfies, they're better protected from snoops and the dark lords of the Internet. Also consider turning off any streaming function on your smartphone that **automatically backs up** pics to the Cloud, which hackers could try to penetrate. And remember! Never show your face (just in case something *should* get in the wrong hands).

My guy wants me to *sext* him a naked pic, but *I don't want to.* What other naughty stuff can I do with *my cell?*

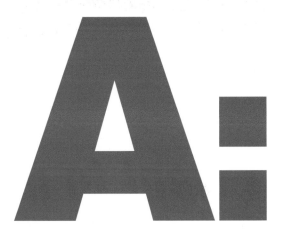

It depends. If you're hesitant to sext him because you're not sure he'll keep the photos private, then that's a red flag that he might not be the right guy for you . . . and you shouldn't send him dirty messages, naked or not. But if that's not the issue and you're more worried about stuff like hacking or showing off your body, then yes, there are tons of hot ways to use your phone. Tease him with pics that show only a hint of your abs, the curve of your hip, or jaw-dropping cleavage. Or try these tamer (but still seductive) options: Send him a pic of the underwear you'll wear that night, or text him a photo of the hot dress you have on and that you can't wait for him to rip it off you later.

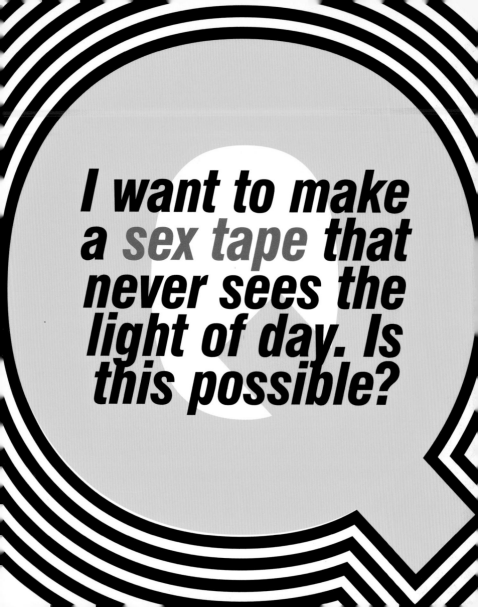

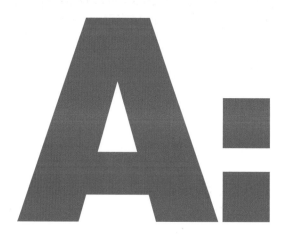

The only way to ensure your grandma never sees your O-face is to delete, delete, delete. Obviously give yourselves an opportunity to enjoy the film before erasing the evidence. Also an option: Bury the flick in a folder within a folder within a folder on your computer, with a boring name that would never intrigue anyone, like Thank-You Card List. If you can save it as a file that's password-protected, that's even better. Extra precaution: When you're filming, keep your faces out of the shot, and cover any birthmarks or tattoos with makeup.

how to talk dirty without sounding ridiculous

WE ALL WANT TO BE that mythical sexy girl who always knows the perfect naughty something to whisper in her guy's ear. But in reality, most of us are stumped as to what sounds hot instead of cheesy or porny. Here are a few sexy pointers to help get the conversation flowing. . . .

1

START SIMPLE. The bedroom doesn't have to be a venue to spout the filthiest thing you can imagine. Phrases as simple as "Oh, that's hot" or "That feels so good" will get temperatures rising.

2

ASK FOR WHAT FEELS GOOD. If you're at a loss for words, tell your partner what hot, dirty things you'd love for him to do. If he's already doing them, tell him how much you enjoy them.

3

TRY A FOUR-LETTER WORD. Experiment with a little swearing in bed. Like a primal scream, you won't know how good an f-bomb feels until you let it out. And your partner will love how worked up you are.

4

STROKE HIS . . . EGO. Don't be afraid to tell your guy everything you like about his body, his penis, or what he does that drives you crazy. He'll be obsessed.

DOES HE REALLY WANT TO HEAR

"YOU'RE SO BIG"

IN BED?

For years, it's been the go-to naughty phrase. Do men still buy it . . . or is it totally clichéd? We polled ninety-nine guys for the verdict.

64% of men say, "IT'S HOT!"

36% of men say, "IT'S A CLICHÉ."

I don't feel comfortable or confident when I attempt to talk dirty during sex. How do I spice things up and try new things without feeling so uncomfortable?

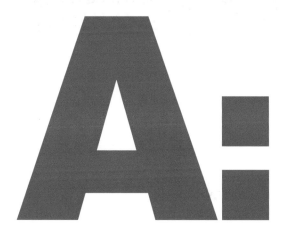

Everyone has different levels of comfort. It's good to know your limits, and it's fun to test them too. That's another bonus of sexting: Consider it practice to get more comfortable with dirty talk. You get to type outrageous things without actually saying them out loud. You can edit what you type. You don't have to see the other person's WTF look if it doesn't click. And you can type things you would never feel comfortable saying in person. After a little playful sexting, you might even, as writers like to say, find your voice.

how to
have HOT
skype sex

Whether your partner's out of town or you're just looking to spice things up, here are six simple steps to having the best (SKYPE) sex of your life.

1 **WRITE IT DOWN.** Before you start, write ten or more things you want to "do" to your partner—role-play, dirty talk, touching, striptease, etc.—and send these saucy tips to each other.

2 **DRESS THE PART.** Don't be afraid to get into it! Pretend like he's there and dress up in some sexy lingerie that really puts you in the mood. Don't forget the sexy music—and keep some lube handy too.

3 **LIGHTEN THE MOOD.** Acknowledge any nerves you have about getting busy over the interwebs. Share a few silly laughs with your guy to lighten the mood. Bonus: Laughing gets the blood flowing and is a turn-on!

4 **JUST BREATHE.** Create some tension by gazing into each other's eyes and breathing deeply via webcam. This heightens anticipation and gets your mind ready for the sexy-times ahead.

5 **GET IN TOUCH WITH YOURSELF.** Touch yourself slowly—either through manual stimulation or with a few sex toys—and tease him with a little peek-a-boo. Instruct him to do a little striptease and masturbation for your viewing pleasure.

6 **LET LOOSE.** You might feel silly at first, but have fun. Video sex has a distinct benefit over sexting or phone sex: You *actually* get to see each other. Pretend like you're in the same room, and after a while, you'll feel as though you're together.

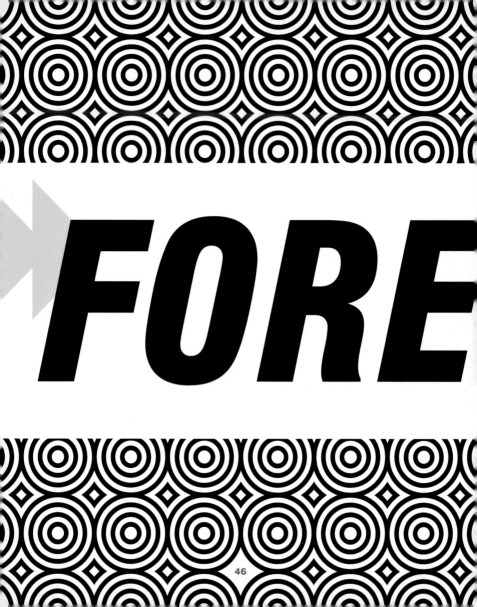

FORE

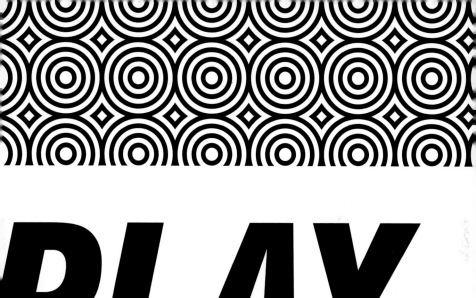

PLAY

Intercourse gets all the glory, but the lead-up should be just as hot as the **MAIN EVENT**. Epic sex starts with great sexpectations—so go forth and **GET BUSY**.

GET INTO THE (EROGENOUS) ZONE ▶▶

Chances are, you and your guy have a few **GO-TO MOVES** that are guaranteed to get you both hot and primed for action. And while it's great that you know what works on your bodies, sticking to the same old thing (an ear nibble here, a nipple lick there) won't lead to a **BED-SHAKING FINALE**.

So, on the hunt for new tricks, we consulted top foreplay experts and discovered **UNCHARTED** erogenous zones so packed with powerful nerve endings that just touching them takes you from 0 to, um, 69.

1 THE ULTRASENSITIVE BORDER AROUND THE LIPS

Okay, so you know how to kiss. But what you probably don't know is that there's an undercover **pleasure** transmitter, the buccal nerve, surrounding the edges of the mouth.

When you're making out, you don't need to lick around his entire mouth to get the **benefits**—that would be weird. Instead, kiss him as you normally do, then use the tip of your tongue to trace the edge of his upper lip lightly. Pull back and **playfully** kiss him again, then trace the border of his bottom lip.

❷ THAT SEXY DIP WHERE NECK MEETS CHEST

As you kiss down his neck, trail the tips of your index and middle fingers from one of his shoulders to the dip in the center, **lingering** to swirl your fingers in a slow, circular motion. Then move your mouth over the spot and kiss it, using your breath to **warm** the area.

❸ THE EROTIC PATHWAYS ON THE SIDES OF THE TORSO

Snaking from the bottom of the rib cage to the hips is a powerful nerve that, when stimulated, **connects** directly to your clitoris and your man's penis.

You'll want to use a firmer touch here, since it's more **ticklish** than other spots. Start on one side, just underneath the rib cage, and either stroke the area with your hand or alternate between kissing (apply more **pressure** than usual with your lips) and lightly nibbling your way down to the hipbone.

4 THE TEASING TRAIL ON THE THIGHS

One of the most explosive nerves in the body is located at the tops of the inner thighs.

In fact, it's best to **save it** for last and work your way up to it. Start by licking your finger (the wetness increases the stimulation) and slowly drawing it from the mid-inner thigh to the top. Then **follow** the path you just traced with your tongue, **teasing** your way to the upper region.

want
CRAZY
romantic
sex?
START HERE . . .

Three foolproof ways to turn up the heat.

1. SURPRISE HIM

When you're in the middle of an innocent conversation, stop midway and tell him how hot you think he is. The unexpectedness—and the fact that you just couldn't hold back—will make him feel amazing, not to mention really turn him on.

2. MAKE HIM WAIT

Once you've gotten physical, keep your underwear on for as long as you both can bear. The anticipation will make you guys want each other that much more.

3. KISS LIKE THIS

Gently suck his upper lip, then his lower one, then go for a deep-kiss kill. A little tongue teasing at first will make your kisses feel more intense.

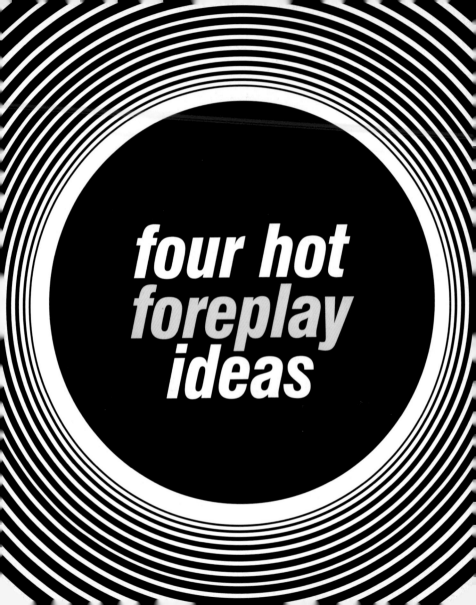

four hot foreplay ideas

1 Formally invite his penis. Tonight, it's all play, no work. Let him know you're flipping the script by sending him the evening itinerary as an iCal (personal e-mail, not work!) invite. Shoot him an appointment for an 8:00 p.m blow-j, then request he return the favor at 8:15. He'll never accept an invite more enthusiastically.

----

2 Make a spicy shopping list. When writing your weekend to-do list, rock his world with a kinky surprise: Right after "pasta and pesto" and "liquor store yay," jot down a superbreezy "cock ring from sex toy store" request. He'll be happy to run home and see what other "favors" he can do for you.

----

3 Do you (while he watches). The best part of waking up—sorry, not sorry, Folgers—is sexual arousal! Hit your own alarm button (you know the one) and make him study every stroke. Task him with re-creating the moves on you tonight, and promise you'll return the favor.

----

4 Shower before! Most people like to shower after sex, but sometimes it's fun to make it part of foreplay. Get some eucalyptus and peppermint oils, and lather up: The combo of scrubbing plus steam will get your blood flowing, so by the time you get to the bed you're extra-energized. Plus, you'll smell nice and feel soft!

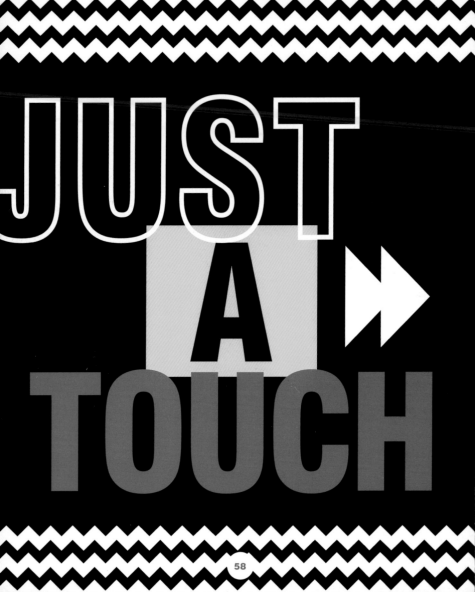

JUST A ▶▶
TOUCH

One perfectly timed brush of the thigh can take a date from pretty good to holy sh*t **THAT'S HOT!** There's a slew of science that proves how the power of touch can **STIR UP** the same kind of sizzle in long-term relationships too. All it takes is knowing a few key moves.

1 SLOW DOWN

Even if you can go from workday to foreplay at the drop of a skirt, it pays to **take your time** doing some necking, as your grandma would say, before you go at it. Run your hands through his hair, kiss his earlobe, and ask him to **rub your back** (don't be surprised if his hands wander).

② GO PANINI STYLE

Make like a human sandwich and lie so you and your guy are both facing down, flat on top of each other, **totally naked.** Let your bodies meld and your breaths sync for a few minutes. The person on top gets to let their limbs go limp and feel the **warmth** of the person underneath. The person on the bottom gets that calm, **secure** feeling you get with a weighted blanket. Plus, your naked bodies smushed together will probably give you a few other ideas. . . .

❸ ZONE IN

His mouth, his nose (yep, we swear), and what he's packing in his boxers are three of his parts most densely populated with nerve endings that connect to the **sensory regions** of the brain. Touch *around* them first, then touch them directly, but not just with your hands—use your lips, tongue, and nipples for **new sensations** that will give him a little thrill.

❹ SHOW AND TELL

Which of your body parts make you feel **sexiest?** (We'll give you a minute to pick just one, you little minx.) Settled? Grab his hands and place them there.

TAKE OFF THE DAMN BRA

5

Sometimes it feels like too much trouble to pull your
T-shirt all the way off and get **stark naked.** But do it.
There's more skin-on-skin contact, which means more
nerves get **stimulated,** which means a stronger orgasm.

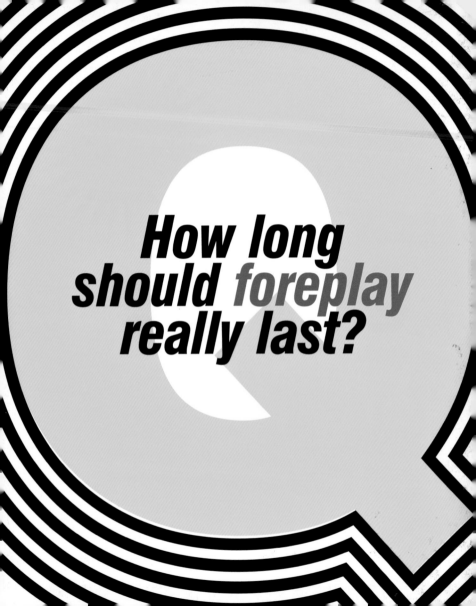

How long should foreplay really last?

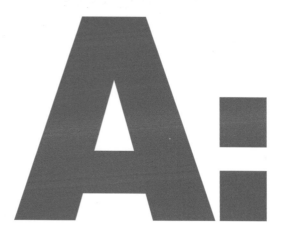

The general rule is about twenty minutes. That number came from a landmark study conducted by Alfred Kinsey in 1953. He found that 92 percent of women orgasm during intercourse if they engage in at least twenty-one minutes of foreplay. When you touch/stroke/kiss for that long, it allows more blood to flow to your genitals, which primes your body for climax. You may require more or less time, and that might even change depending on how horny you are at that moment. Bottom line: While this info is good to keep in mind, you should focus on the sensations you're experiencing, not meeting a specific time goal.

getting it on

okay, you're warmed up. you're in the mood.

All you need is a partner and ideally forty, but let's face it, even fifteen minutes of privacy and you're ready to **go-go-OH!** In this chapter, we've mapped out all the basics, from giving (and, most important, **getting**) the best oral of your life, to artful and fun **twists** on all the basic positions. You may think you've had good sex before, but **stick with us, kid:** You're about to have the best. Sex. Ever.

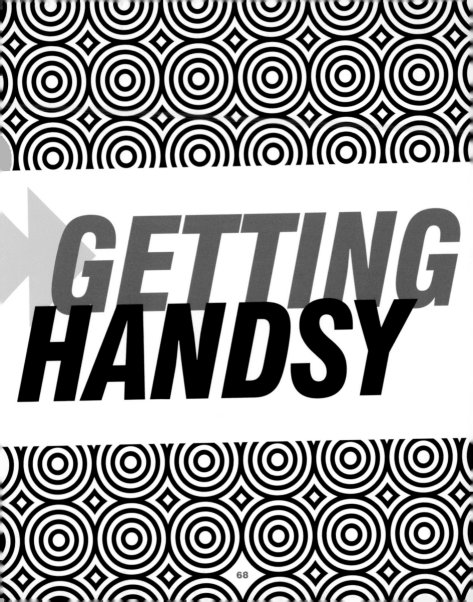

GETTING HANDSY

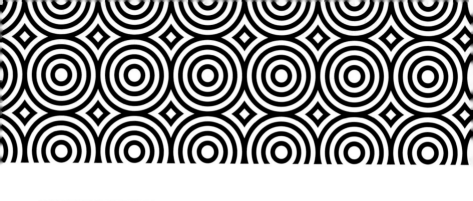

HAND JOBS get a bad rap as a move that's rarely revisited after high school. But say good-bye to the jerky HJ! These pleasurable moves will show you how to give a hand job like a **GROWN-UP** and leave him dreaming about first base.

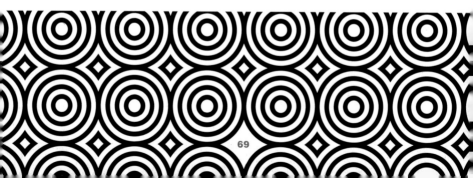

HANDY
HAND
JOB ▶▶
TIPS

1 GRIP HIM FIRMLY.

If your grasp is **too tight,** he'll let you know.

2 USE LUBE (OR SPIT).

Wet both palms and gently twist them as you move up and down his shaft. Ask him to put his hand over yours and show you how he likes to be **touched**—after all, he's probably given himself a hand job or two in his day.

BEGINNER

the love tunnel

Place one hand over the other again and again and push them down from the head to the base, which makes him feel like he's in a **never-ending** vagina.

the sausage wrap

To nail this classic handy technique, **wrap** all your fingers around him and stroke up and down. Then try the Reverse Sausage Wrap: Turn your hand upside down (so your thumb is toward the base of his penis instead of the tip). It's a **totally different** feeling for him.

INTERMEDIATE

the sexy squid

Put your hand in a squid shape with all your fingers pursed together around the tip of his penis, your palm above the head. Now **bounce** it up and down his penis from the head to the base, trying to get the thumb or middle finger to go down over the frenulum (on the underside of his penis, just below the head) **repeatedly**.

TRY THIS
Changing up the angle of your body will affect what he feels, so vary your position. Sit to one side, on top of him, or stand behind him and reach your hand around.

the **windshield wiper**

Do the Sausage Wrap, but every time you reach the top of his penis, **swipe** your thumb to one side of the head and then the other, like a miniature windshield wiper.

ADVANCED

the **DIY penis ring**

Make the A-OK sign and squeeze the base of his **magic wand** with that hand. (Use a good, solid grip. It acts like a penis ring to trap blood, making him harder and more sensitive to your touch.) Now **slide** your other hand up and down his penis.

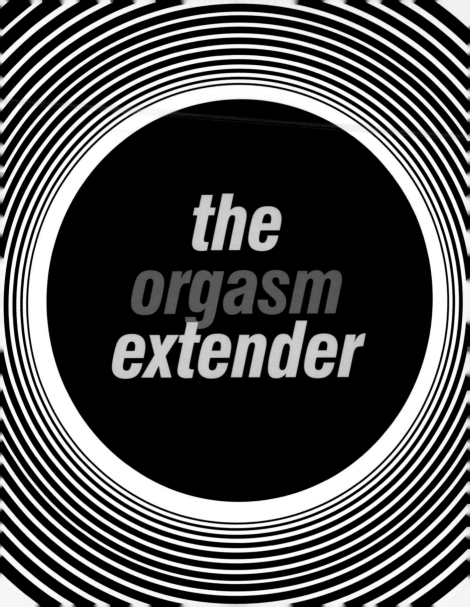

the orgasm extender

Two of the biggest hand job mistakes that women make happen at the very end.

1 Maintain a steady grip and rhythm, even if you feel he's about to climax. Only change things up at that point if you're trying to make him last longer.

2 Don't let go too soon. A man's orgasm can last for several seconds, and it feels awesome for him if you're pumping the whole time. If you release your hand right when he comes, it's a buzzkill. Wait for him to give you the cue that he's done.

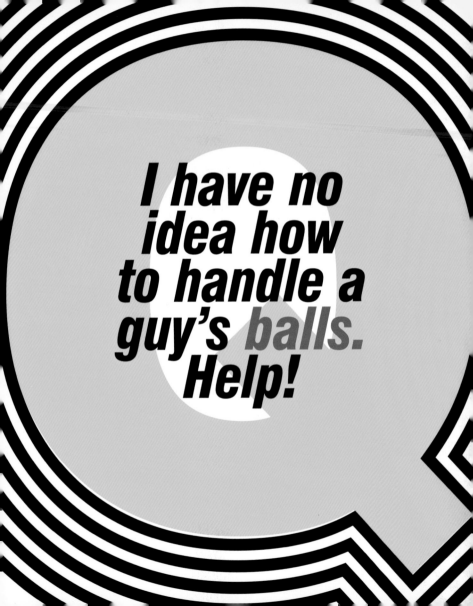

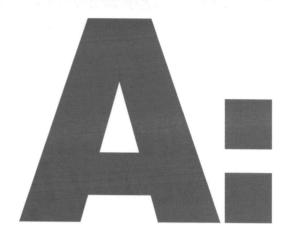

Delicately . . . to start, at least! First, cup his
jewels in one hand while you run your other
hand up and down his shaft or go down on
him. Once he's turned on, he can withstand
more pressure. Try gently tugging on his balls
or massaging them with the palm of your
hand while you're on top of him. Now go out
there and grab his balls by the balls!

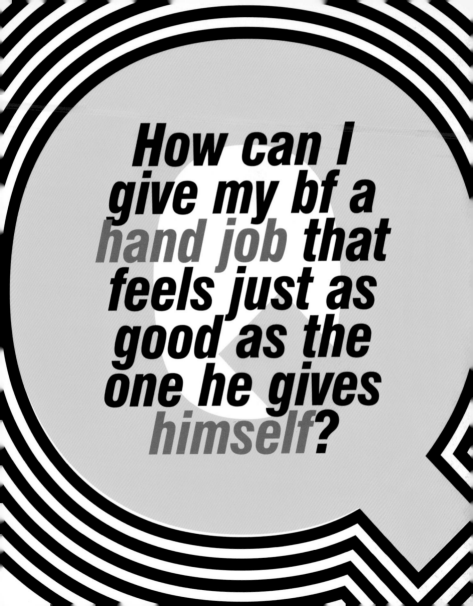

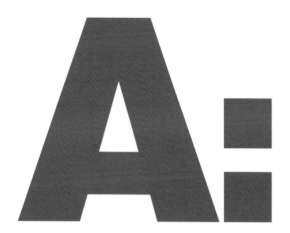

A:

Ask him to show you what he likes. If he's not comfortable (or you aren't) masturbating in front of you, have him put his hand over yours while you touch him. That way you can feel what kind of grip and speed he prefers. Also, ask if he likes any extras—many men cup or stroke their scrotum. Not dating the vocal type? Experiment with touches and speeds, and pay attention to his reactions—quickened breath, tense muscles, and red flush all indicate he's enjoying what you're doing.

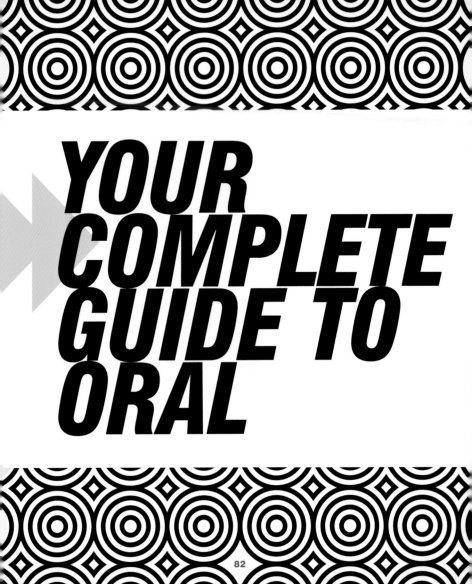

YOUR COMPLETE GUIDE TO ORAL

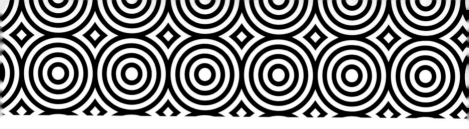

Stuff we feel NEUTRAL about: Chicken pot pie. *Dancing with the Stars.* Woodchucks. But one thing you shouldn't have a take-it-or-leave-it attitude toward is TONGUE ACTION. Oral is the form of sex that the majority of women say is most likely to give them an ORGASM. Get ready to get—and give—the best oral of your life.

OUR
TURN ▶▶

GET
YOURSELF
GOING

1 If you're self-conscious **about the way you smell or taste (and you shouldn't be!!), take a shower or use a wet wipe beforehand.**

---

2 Close your eyes **if it helps you turn off your brain.**

---

3 Show your partner with your hand **where you want to be touched and the kinds of motions you like.**

---

4 Don't forget to show your appreciation, **whether it's through moans, body language, or the very straightforward "Yes!" (Your partner will appreciate the positive feedback!)**

BEGINNER

the human vibrator

Have your partner **moan or hum** while he goes down on you. ("Babe, this is gonna sound weird, but humor me. . . ." is a good way to intro the topic.) Yeah, humming while giving oral sex might seem kind of goofy at first, but the vibrations will feel **so good**, you'll soon be drowning it out with noises of your own.

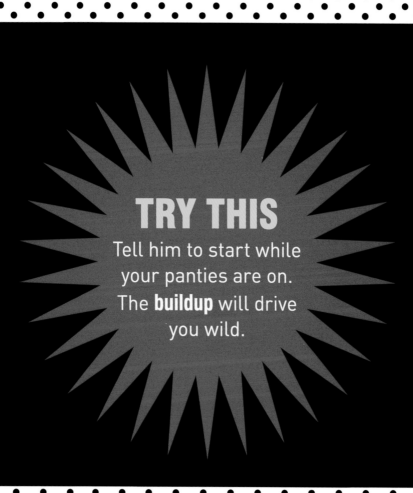

TRY THIS

Tell him to start while your panties are on. The **buildup** will drive you wild.

INTERMEDIATE

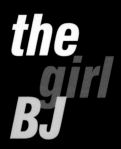

the girl BJ

This is when a guy gently pulls your clit into his mouth, **sucking and swirling** with his tongue. Have him start gently, and then gradually amp up the intensity.

ADVANCED

G marks the spot

Have him stroke your **G-spot** with his finger while he uses his tongue on your clitoris. You can show him how to reach your G-spot by demonstrating a palms-up "come hither" **motion** with your index finger.

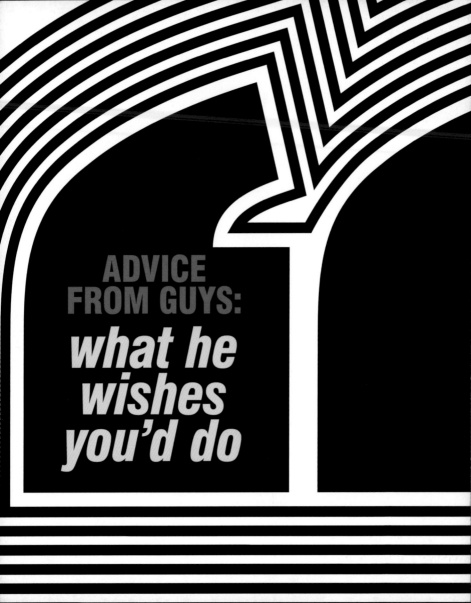

ADVICE
FROM GUYS:
*what he
wishes
you'd do*

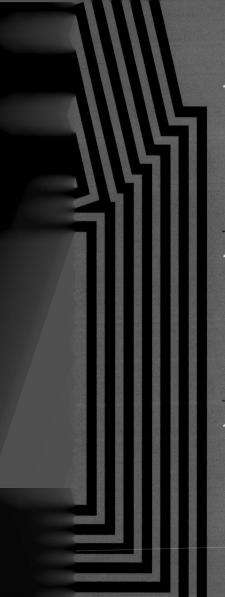

"When I'm giving you oral, put one hand on the back of my head and press me closer to you, and at the same time, push up with your hips. It lets me know you're into what I'm doing."—**IAN W.**

"Tell me what you want me to do with my hands while I'm going down on you. Say where you want me to touch you, or better yet, put my hands exactly where you want them."—**JOHN T.**

"Mid sex, while you're on top, make your way up to my head and kneel over my face so I can perform oral while you hold on to the bed frame."—**MAX W.**

My boyfriend is totally clueless when going downtown on me. How can I give him a quick lesson without bruising his ego?

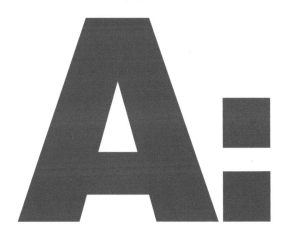

A:

When a man is tending to your delicate flower, his ego can be a delicate flower too. Start with positive feedback, and then segue to what you really want. Something like "Mmm, that feels so great. Could you go a little harder?" (Feel free to swap *harder* for *faster, softer,* or *slower.*) Cat got your tongue? Reach down and gently adjust the position of his face or hand. Once he gets it right, tell him to keep doing exactly what he's doing and to pretty much never stop. He'll be a pro in no time.

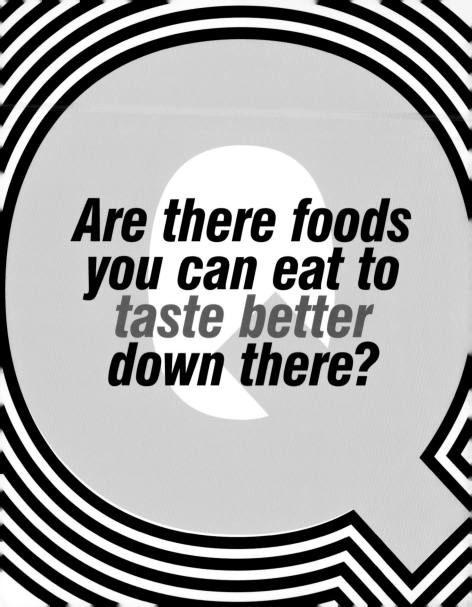

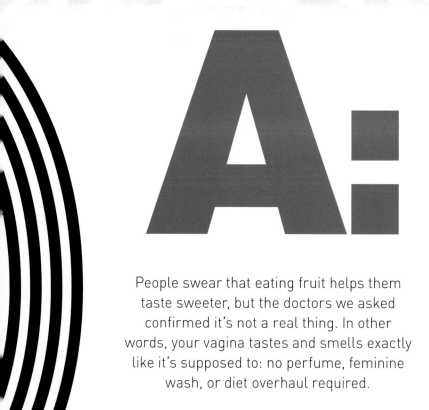

People swear that eating fruit helps them taste sweeter, but the doctors we asked confirmed it's not a real thing. In other words, your vagina tastes and smells exactly like it's supposed to: no perfume, feminine wash, or diet overhaul required.

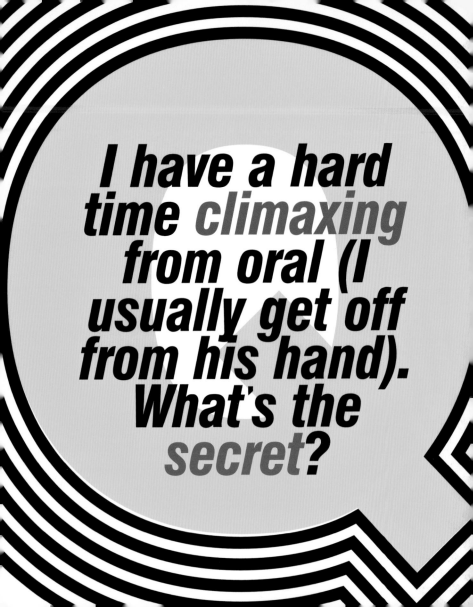

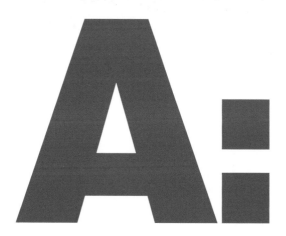

You know what works for you manually, so have him use the same pressure and motion with his mouth. For example, if you like constant, firm contact with the palm of his hand, have him purse his lips, press them firmly against you, and move in circles, up and down, etc. Or if you prefer a lighter touch with his fingertips, ask him to tease your clitoris gently with the tip of his tongue. And have him use his hands—he can caress your thighs, pubic mound, and breasts.

HIS TURN ▸▸

GET HIM GOING

Here's the basic rule to giving a great blow job: Use your mouth (obviously) and your hands. Your mouth is going to provide the sensation (and for him, an all-important visual), but your hands are going to do a lot of the work. So for a starter blow job, try this: Take the head into your mouth and **squeeze, lick, and swirl** like you would a soft-serve cone. Meanwhile, use your hands to grip, squeeze, and stroke the length of his penis. Don't just keep doing the same motion—variety of sensation is key!

BEGINNER

the tip-off

The hole on his tip is called the meatus, which is the worst name given to anything, ever.

(MEATUS!)

But it's **sensitive** during arousal.

With your tongue, apply medium pressure, on and off. It might sound crazy, but rest assured, pleasuring it will feel crazy to him too. He'll be shocked it **feels so good!**

INTERMEDIATE

ice, ice baby

Alternating hot and cold **sensations** really does feel amazing for him. If you're too lazy for the ol' ice-cube-in-the cheek trick (or if your teeth are too sensitive), try alternating oral with drinking something cold or warm. Even easier: **Lightly blow** air over him after having had him in your mouth.

ADVANCED

the
corkscrew

Twist your hand as you move up and down his shaft like you're tracing the grooves of a **corkscrew** and slide it over his tip when you get to it.

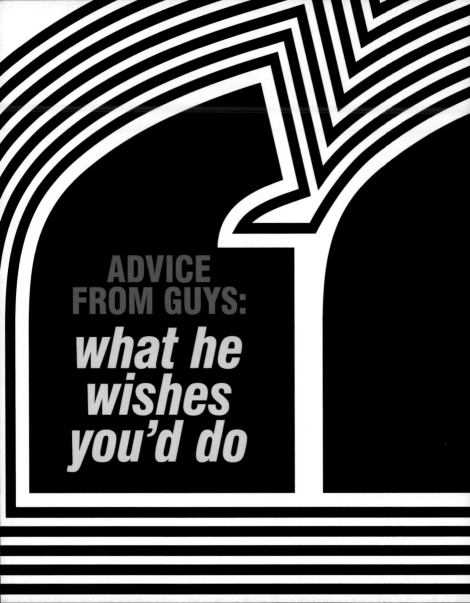

ADVICE
FROM GUYS:
*what he
wishes
you'd do*

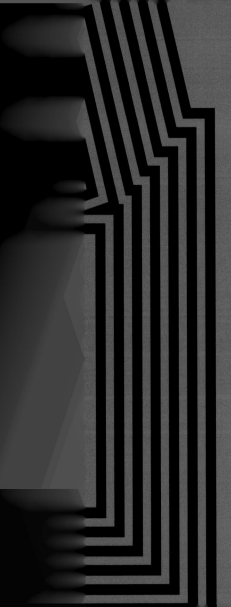

"I love a little ball-massage action during oral. Gently rub my scrotum and apply some pressure to the muscle under my balls. It'll make me go nuts—pun intended."
—WARREN J.

"It's hot when a girl tells me when and where to climax. But it's even more of a turn-on if you say something like 'I can't wait to taste. . .' Deep down, guys know semen isn't appetizing, so we love it when you make us feel like it's the best thing ever."**—ANDY H.**

"The hand is an underrated and underused part of a good blow job. There isn't nearly enough friction in the mouth alone, so the extra attention is amazing. A little firmness goes a long way."**—AMAN G.**

finishing
MANEUVERS

**Figure out what to do
with the semen ahead of time,
or at least partway through,
during a break in the action.**

Our survey respondents
said they swallow:

27% Every Time
34% Never
32% Sometimes

If swallowing isn't your thing, spit or ask
him to finish someplace else
(your body? the bed? an old-timey spittoon?).
Whatever works for you!

MIND-BLOWING

oral sex

POSITIONS

Use these hot oral sex positions as foreplay or as the main event. No rules here!

the
cliffhanger

Sit with your butt on the edge of the bed and then lay back with your legs draped over the edge. When he **kneels** on the floor between your legs, his head will be angled down toward your vagina, giving him direct access to your clitoris. This one also leaves his hands **free to play** with your nipples or finger you for double pleasure.

doggy goes oral

Not only is this a totally hot oral position that puts **you in control** of the angle and pressure, it's also a good segue into the world of anilingus (which is exactly what it sounds like), if that's something you're into.

the sidecar

Lie on your sides facing each other, then slide down until his penis is, well, in your face. Call it the lazy woman's blow job. This position is the best way to give him **pleasure** without killing your knees or getting a major neck cramp, and you can also get saucy by **reaching around** to play with his back door.

the so-fa
so good

Have your guy lie upside down on the couch, with his back and head on the seat and his legs draped over the back. **Kneel** over his face, facing the back of the couch. Then bend over and 69 away. Much more **relaxing** than an awkward, limb-flailing 69 in bed, isn't it?

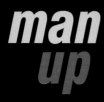

man up

While girl-on-top 69 has its advantages—you get to be the one in control—this twist is a **hot way** to change it up and give your man a few new thrills. It's a very gratifying spot for him to be in—he has you pinned down and is also **in charge** of the depth and pace. However this does not give him a free pass to jackhammer your face. Agree on a safety signal, like pinching his thigh, if he gets too carried away.

too naughty to name

If you and your guy are feeling **adventurous**, here's a challenge: Have him sit on the couch, his legs stretched out and slightly parted, knees bent, and feet resting on a hard surface, like a coffee table. Stand behind the couch and, leaning over, place your elbows on either side of his hips as you **lower your head** between his thighs. With the majority of your weight supported by your elbows, place your knees on the back of the couch, so you're straddling his face. Yeah, it's **acrobatic**, but that's half the fun.

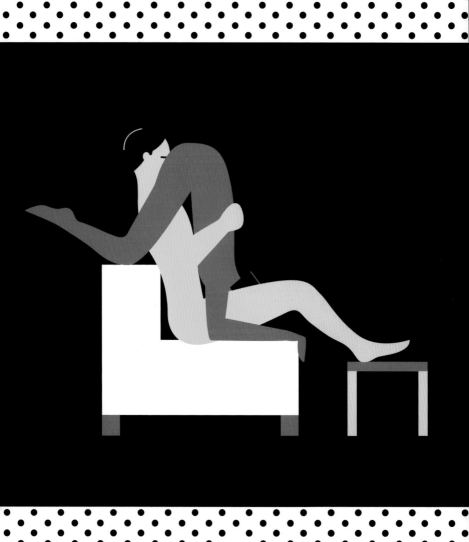

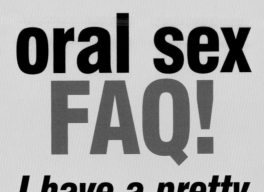

oral sex
FAQ!

I have a pretty sensitive gag reflex. What can I do to make giving my boyfriend oral easier?

LOTS OF WOMEN HAVE THIS ISSUE. It's because we didn't Darwinianly adapt to being able to take penises deep into our throats. No matter! Just take in as much as you can handle and fake the rest, using your hands. Or, you can try lying on your side (à la 69), which opens up the pathway in your throat. Remember, it's varied pressure and warmth that make him feel good, not your tonsils.

ANYTHING I CAN DO TO AVOID TMJ?

The blow job jaw ache *sucks* (pun intended), but luckily there are some pretty easy fixes. Aching jaws tend to happen when we open our mouths too wide or make a repetitive motion for too long, so do yourself a favor and mix it up down there. There are lots of things you can do during oral besides sucking (like licking and kissing, not just the shaft but his balls, thighs, etc.) that make for a very sexy break.

KISSING AFTER ORAL: GROSS? HOT? WHAT'S THE NORM HERE?

This is completely up to you and your partner! In terms of hygiene or health, if it's safe to perform oral on each other, then kissing after is safe too. As for whether to do it, that's just a matter of personal preference. Whatever you're into, rest assured that it's perfectly normal.

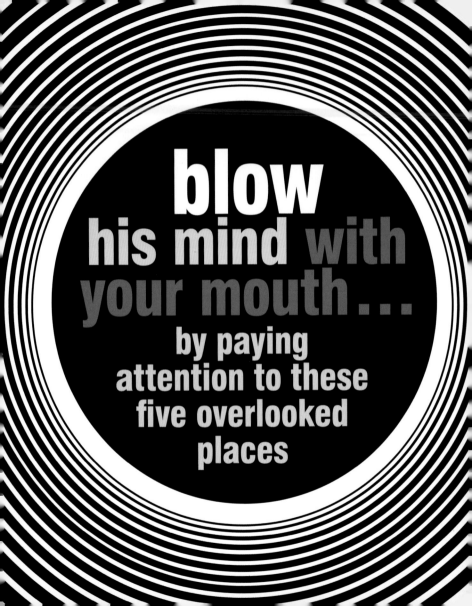

1 His hipbones: Run your lips along his hipbones while slowly making your way toward his package. There are a ton of nerve endings there that are craving more attention.

2 His balls: The next time you give your man downstairs action, keep this *Cosmo* fact in mind: Most men feel their balls are ignored during foreplay. Be the girl who reads his mind by lightly sucking where he wants it most.

3 His pubic mound: While running your mouth down his chest, stop to kiss and nip around his pubic mound. Just like yours, it's an overlooked hot spot.

4 The area where the scrotum meets the perineum: This spot is ultrasensitive. Press on it with your tongue. His erectile tissue extends all the way back there, so it'll give him a jolt of pleasure.

5 The frenulum: Keep your tongue stiff as you slide it back and forth over his frenulum (remember: that's the underside of the penis where the head meets the shaft), or cover your teeth with your lips and lightly nibble on it.

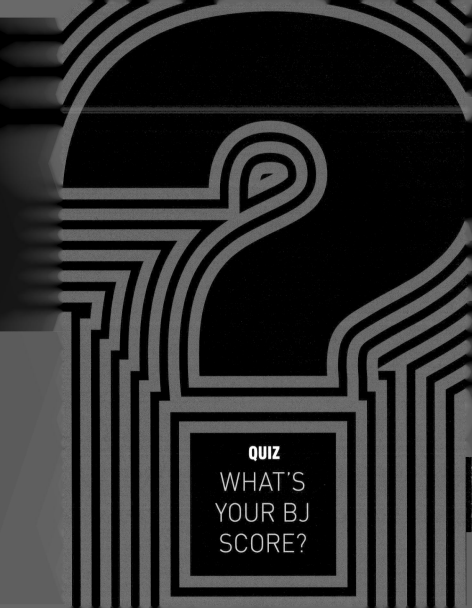

QUIZ

WHAT'S
YOUR BJ
SCORE?

Ever wake him up with surprise oral?

a. All the time. Yeah, he loves me.
b. He might get lucky on our anniversary or something.
c. No way, things are stank in the morning.

When your mouth gets tired, you:

a. Switch to a good old-fashioned hand job, occasionally licking the tip.
b. Take a ten-second breather.
c. Stop and initiate regular sex instead.

Balls?

a. Of course, they're part of the deal. Lick, suck, tug . . . all for it.
b. I'll sort of cup them with one hand, but only his penis gets near my mouth.
c. I pretty much ignore the twins, to be perfectly honest.

Any extras?

a. I stroke his perineum with my hand and give him a lot of eye contact.
b. I moan loudly and add a lot of *Mmm*s, so he feels the vibration on his penis.
c. Nada—He's lucky I'm down there to begin with.

MOSTLY As: A FOR ADVANCED

Dear Lord, woman, we bow in your presence! Just make sure he returns the favor.

MOSTLY Bs: B FOR BASIC

Nothing wrong with your skills, but you could push the boundaries and experiment a little more. Amp it up from time to time—remember, it's not about just the penis.

MOSTLY Cs: C FOR . . . COME ON, REALLY?

He's not going to complain; a BJ is a BJ. But you're obviously only doing it because you feel like you should—and we bet he knows it. Try having more fun with it—for his sake and yours.

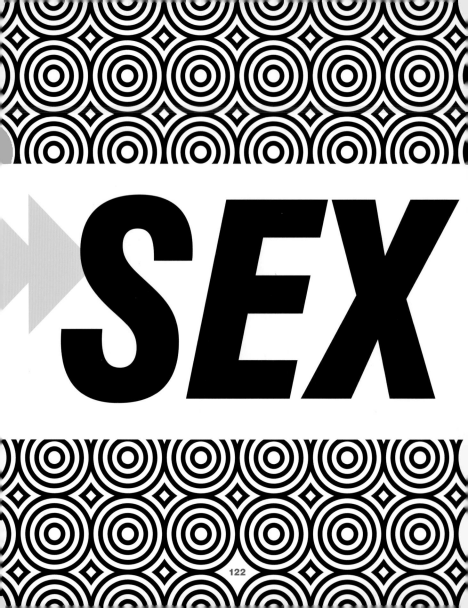

SEX

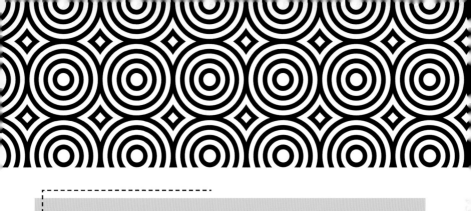

Great sex is about confidence in yourself and your moves, and **ENTHUSIASM**, whether it's missionary or trying out an ambitious sex position that you don't **QUITE** have the hang of yet. Oh, and one more thing: **PRACTICE**. And that's where the real fun begins. . . .

the most important sex tip in this book: love your body

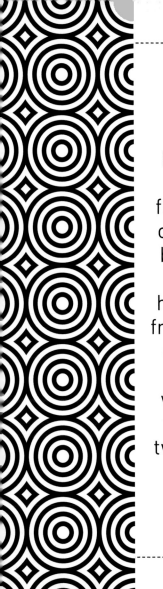

LOOK AT YOURSELF naked in a full-length mirror for five minutes a day and focus on what you love about your body. If this feels awkward, get ready or blow out your hair while standing naked in front of the mirror. By getting used to your unique shape, you'll gain confidence that will naturally spill over into your sex life and make you twice as enticing to your guy.

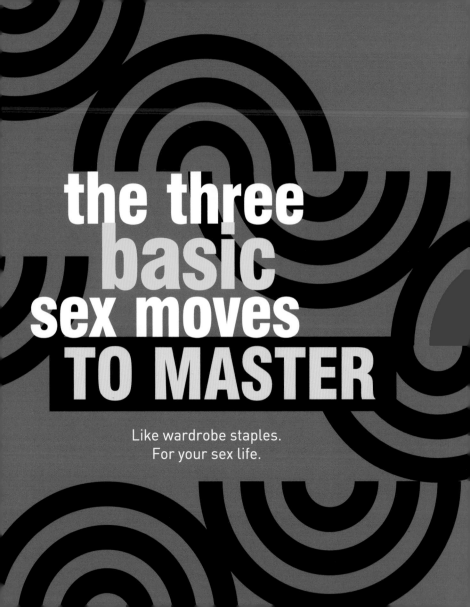

the three basic sex moves
TO MASTER

Like wardrobe staples.
For your sex life.

THE FIGURE EIGHT

Lie on the floor **faceup** with a couple of pillows propping your butt. Keep your knees half bent, your legs splayed wide, and your arms high over your head or holding on to his side (as in the picture) so that your body is **extremely open**. Have your partner enter you at a higher angle than usual (the pillows will help), planting his hands on the floor beside your head. He should move inside you with slow, **languid** figure-eight motions, so that you feel his whole package—his penis plus pubic region. Remember: The figure-eight motion is key to this maneuver.

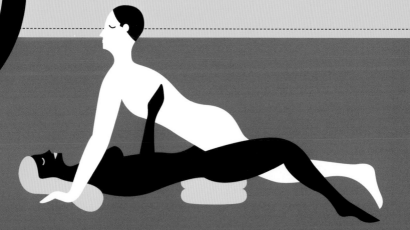

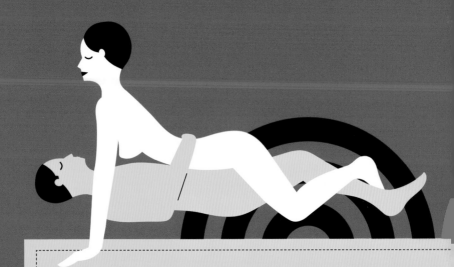

THE RIDE OF YOUR LIFE

Your guy lies on his back. Facing him, lower yourself onto his penis in a kneeling position. Keeping your knees on the bed, curl your feet around the inside of his legs, likely around his knees. **Lean forward** and grab the bedsheets on either side of his head. While holding the sheets—and your feet wrapped around your man's calves—squeeze your butt, **tilt your pelvis**, and move in small, tight motions.

THE LUMBERJACK

Imagine leaning against a tree (or, more realistically, your bedroom wall) and facing him, **lift one leg** and wrap it around his body while he holds the trunk (wall!) for balance. Bonus: This position is an **excellent workout** for your thighs.

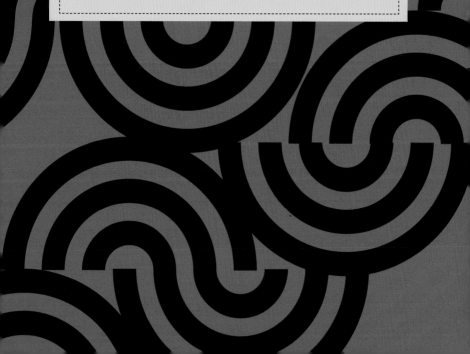

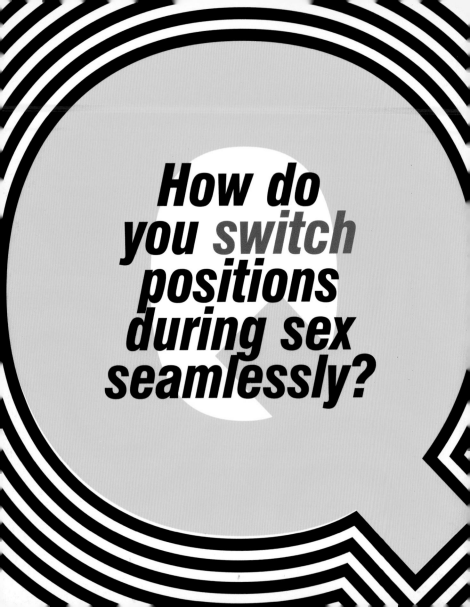

How do you switch positions during sex seamlessly?

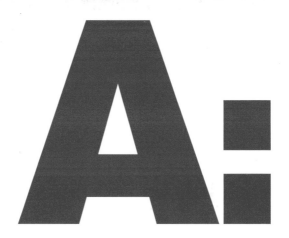

The key is to pick positions that make a switch as easy as possible. First, try missionary to girl-on-top: Entwine your legs in his, then have him pull you up and flip you over. Second, try girl-on-top to missionary: Have him grab you around the waist, then hug each other tightly as you flip over. Third, go from side-by-side to doggy style. When you're the little spoon, turn onto your stomach and have him get on all fours and enter you from behind that way instead.

making the ▶▶ most out of
MISSIONARY

Most of us are fans of the missionary position. And it's no surprise, considering that man-on-top mode is totally intimate, allowing you and your guy constant eye contact and easy access to kissing. Plus it's relatively relaxing for you, putting him in control as you lie back and enjoy.

BEGINNER

a little enthusiasm

If you're kind of shy in bed, try digging your nails into your partner's butt while you're having missionary sex to **pull him closer.** It's an easy way to show how into it you are without shouting!

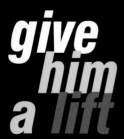

give him a lift

Put both legs up on his shoulders and lift your butt a couple inches off the mattress making it easier for him to go super deep. Then, have your guy **thrust extra hard**. The end result is mind-blowing.

TERMEDIATE

reach for
the heavens

Choose an immovable surface—a **strong headboard** or the side of a tub if you have a spacious bathroom. Lie on your back and raise your arms overhead so your palms rest flat on your surface of choice with your head several inches from the tub or the headboard; it's as if you're reaching for the **sexual stars**. Once he enters you missionary style, bring your legs together as close as possible. With your thighs pressed tightly, his penis will rub against your inner thighs and labia each time he thrusts.

the *soft* rock

Try this **tantalizing twist** on the typical missionary position. Instead of having your man rest on his elbows, ask him to slide two to four inches forward. Have him place his arms on either side of your shoulders, letting his body fall flat against yours. Make sure you both keep your spines straight. With your legs touching his, **push your pelvis** up about two inches. Your man should push down gently, providing a little counter-resistance. Instead of the usual in-and-out of thrusting, rock up and down.

ADVANCED

the passion propeller

Your man lies on top of you, entering you in traditional missionary style, but then—**yowza!**—he starts doing a 360-degree spin, all the while keeping his penis deep inside of you. As he's rotating and thrusting, help guide him around your body like a propeller would **spin around** the top of a helicopter. Make sure to lift his legs when they swing around over your head.

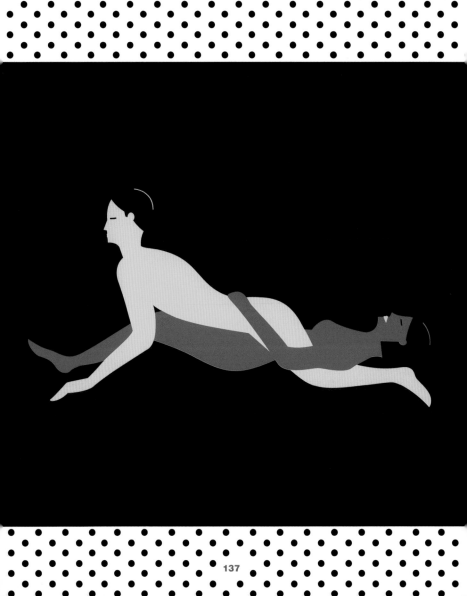

purr-fect position

There's something called the Coital Alignment Technique (CAT), and many sexperts say it's the most **mutually arousing** position of them all. Imagine your body is a surfboard and your man is lying on it, stomach down. From there, have him move a few inches up your body so that his penis, which usually points up, is now pointing down (toward the entrance of your vagina). Once you're in position, start having sex that way, with your guy thrusting down and inward, then up and outward. This provides a **powerful physical connection** plus major clitoral stimulation. Rock back and forth, and enjoy riding the waves.

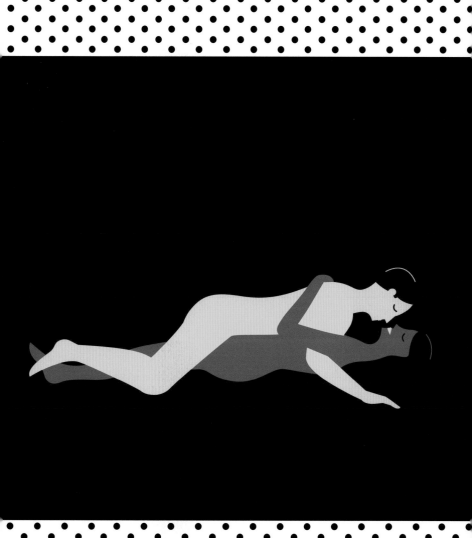

THE COSMO ▶▶
guide to
GIRL ON TOP

It's our favorite position: in bed, at work . . . pretty much everywhere. Why do it lying down, when you can hop up and take control! Grabbing hold of the randy reins may just be the key to your next greatest orgasm.

Your guy probably wants it because he'll get to see you in all your full-frontal glory, a major turn-on for any hot-blooded male. Plus, since he'll have a limited range of motion, he's likely to last longer too. But there are also some sexy advantages for you. This position puts you in control of the pace, motion, and depth of penetration, so you can get the kind of stimulation you need to send you over the edge.

To assume the woman-on-top position, have your guy lie on his back and straddle him with your knees on either side of his hips. Or, if you prefer, you can squat over him with your feet flat on the mattress. Tease him before he enters you by slowly running your fingers down his chest to his shaft and stroking his member till it's good 'n' hard. Then, with one hand on the bed or on his chest for support, hold the base of his penis with your other hand and slowly lower yourself onto him.

Start moving up and down to build momentum. Or you can rest your torso on his and sensuously grind him from side to side or in circles. But just because you're in the driver's seat, that doesn't mean you have to do all the work. To keep from tuckering out, have him wrap his hands around your hips and help you gyrate.

BEGINNER

couch canoodle

Have your partner sit back on a couch (or a comfy chair). **Straddle** his lap with your legs splayed apart and your knees bent up against his chest. Slowly lean back so you're almost upside down with your arms stretched behind you (all the way to the floor) to support your weight and **maintain your balance**. Thrust back and forth against him, opening and closing your legs.

INTERMEDIATE

the erotic end

Sit your lover on the floor with his legs stretched out comfortably in front of him. Have him lean back slightly, using his arms to support his weight. With your back to him and your legs **straddling** his thighs, lower yourself onto him. Keep your knees bent and your feet planted on the floor. With your groins grinding together, **squeeze** your PC (pubococcygeus) muscles (the same ones you squeeze to stop peeing) while he makes small circular rotations with his pelvis.

supernova

Begin in the deceptively down-to-earth woman-on-top position on a made bed. (Don't get under the covers.) But instead of **riding** him with his body lengthwise on the mattress, mount your man as he lies parallel to the pillows— you'll see why in a second. Once you're climbing toward **climax**, stop moving and gently grab the sides of his torso with your hands. Leaning on your knees, inch him toward the edge of the bed until his head, shoulders, and arms hang backward over the side. Then start riding him again.

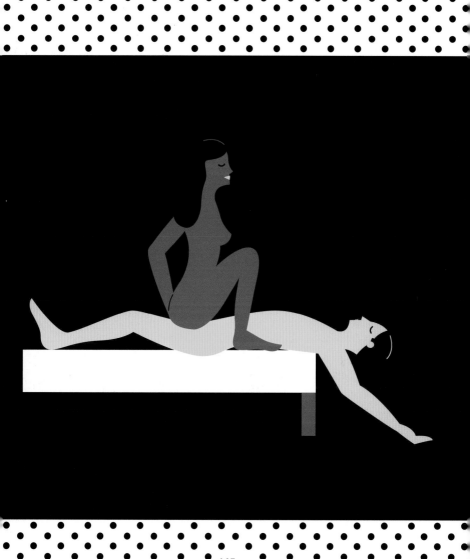

the reverse 50

With him lying on his back, tie his wrists to the bedpost with your panties, bathrobe belt or a pair of **fuzzy handcuffs**. Lower yourself onto him, **straddling** his hips. Have him raise his knees halfway toward his chest so that your thighs hug his in the snuggest possible fit. Now you're in total control!

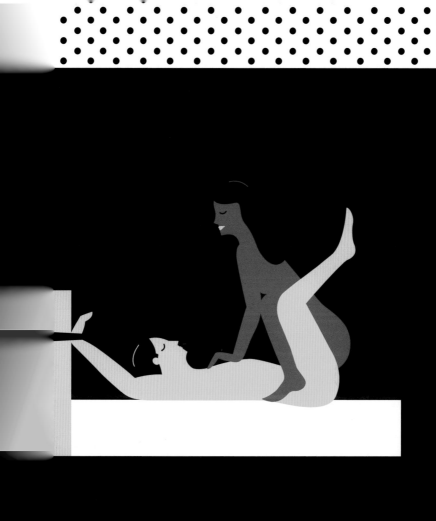

ADVANCED

the octopus

Have your guy sit on the floor with his hands on the ground behind him. Tell him to **spread his legs** and bend them slightly at the knees. Keeping your hands on the floor for support, straddle his lap, facing him, and raise your legs so your right leg rests on his left shoulder and your left leg on his right shoulder. Do it right and you two will look like a multilimbed **lust creature**.

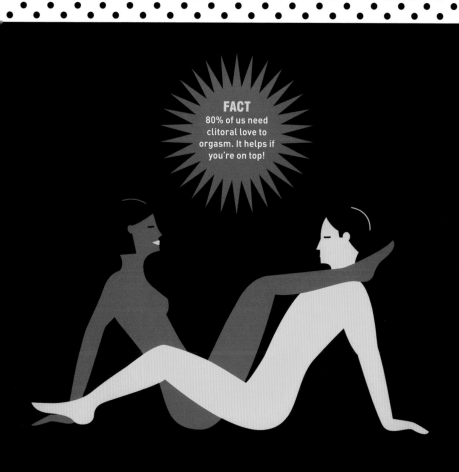

girl on top
FAQ!

I'm a tiny *nymph* who is cowgirling Paul Bunyan. Instead of looking into his eyes, I'm staring directly into . . . his *nipples*. What do I do?

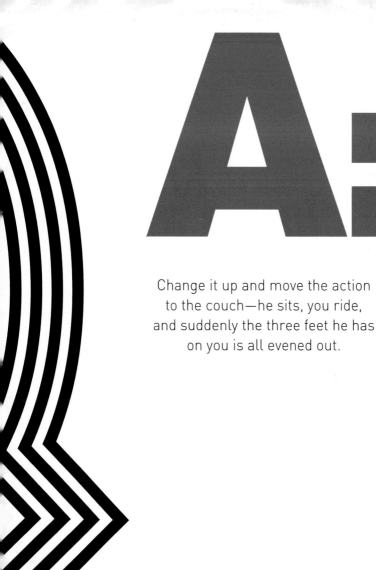

Change it up and move the action to the couch—he sits, you ride, and suddenly the three feet he has on you is all evened out.

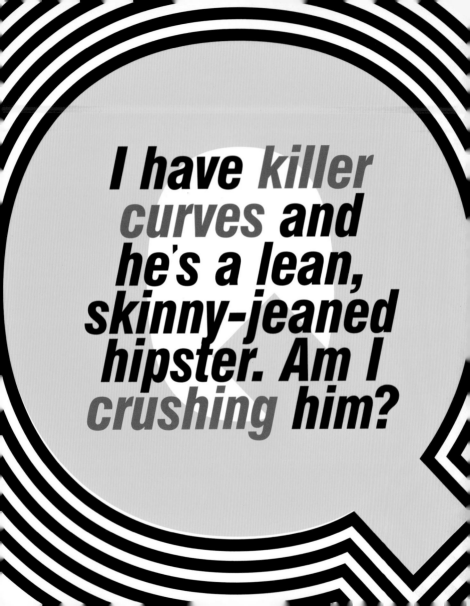

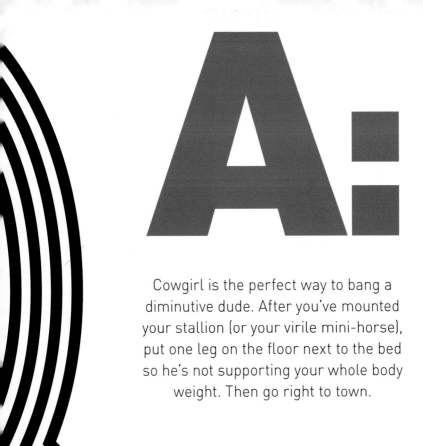

Cowgirl is the perfect way to bang a diminutive dude. After you've mounted your stallion (or your virile mini-horse), put one leg on the floor next to the bed so he's not supporting your whole body weight. Then go right to town.

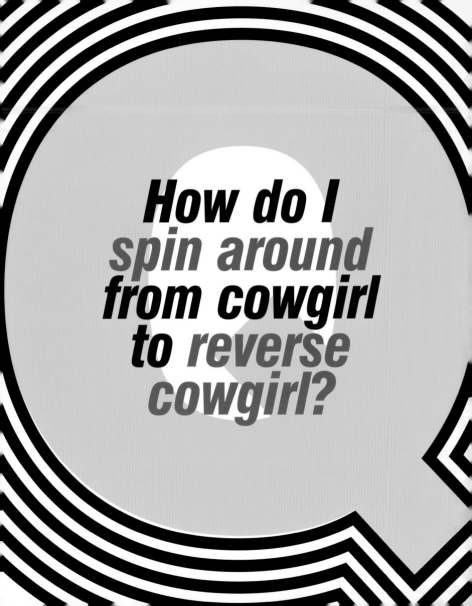

How do I spin around from cowgirl to reverse cowgirl?

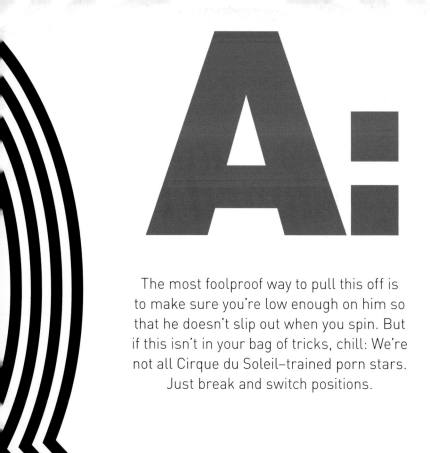

A:

The most foolproof way to pull this off is to make sure you're low enough on him so that he doesn't slip out when you spin. But if this isn't in your bag of tricks, chill: We're not all Cirque du Soleil–trained porn stars. Just break and switch positions.

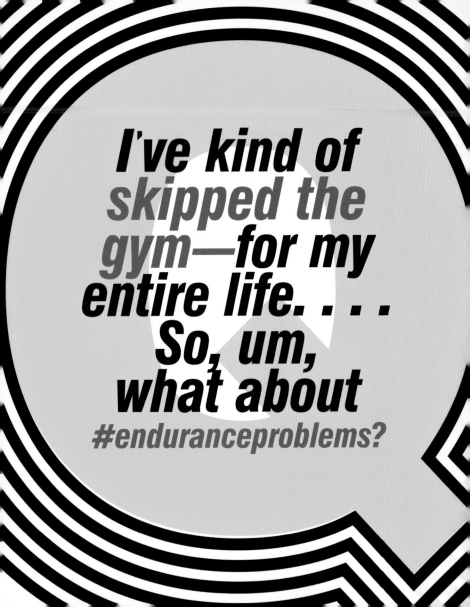

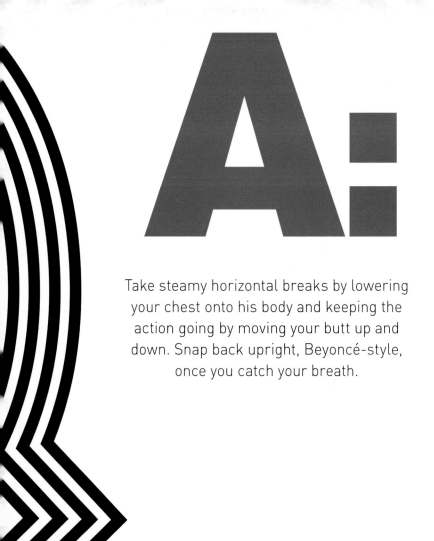

A:

Take steamy horizontal breaks by lowering your chest onto his body and keeping the action going by moving your butt up and down. Snap back upright, Beyoncé-style, once you catch your breath.

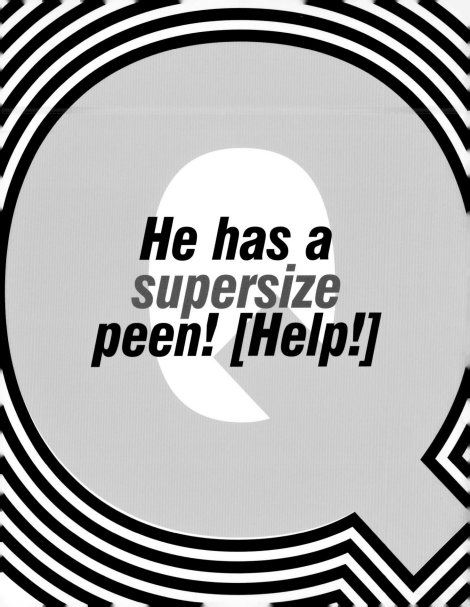

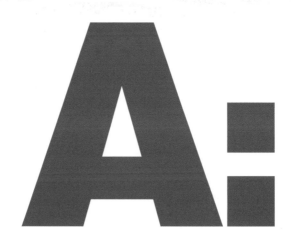

If you're already lubing up (please say you are), just take as much of him as you can handle. The outer third of a woman's vagina is the most sensitive, and he'll like shallow thrusting because it works the head of his penis. And remember, when you're on top you can control his depth of penetration.

SEXY SIDE-BY-SIDES ▶▶

With the benefits of novel nooky in mind, we've mapped out some daring and innovative side-by-side sex positions.

BEGINNER

saucy *spoons*

Lie on your sides with him behind you so you're both facing the same direction. Push your butt toward him as he enters you. Put your hand on his and show him **how you want** your clitoris to be touched. Have him alternate between there and your breasts.

INTERMEDIATE

the linguini

Lie on your side, putting a pillow under your head for **extra support**. Your man kneels directly behind your butt, leaning ever-so-slightly over your body. He should push one of his knees between your legs, positioning his body so he can penetrate you. He places one hand on your back to help support himself as he goes for the plunge. The key to your **pleasure** is keeping your limbs as limp as noodles.

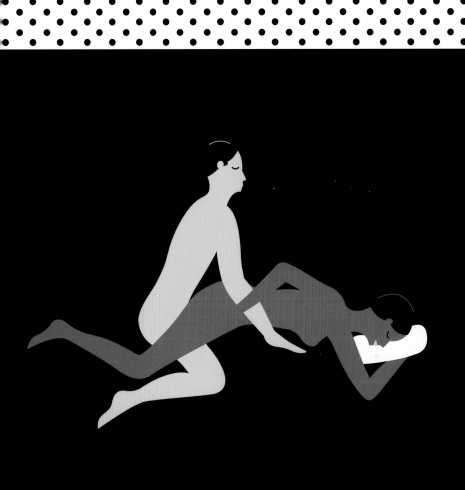

ADVANCED

the spider web

Both you and your guy lie on your sides, facing each other. Lean in close together and **scissor** your legs through his so you're superclose. When he enters you, he'll be deep inside you. While **thrusting**, hold on to each other for leverage and ultimate friction.

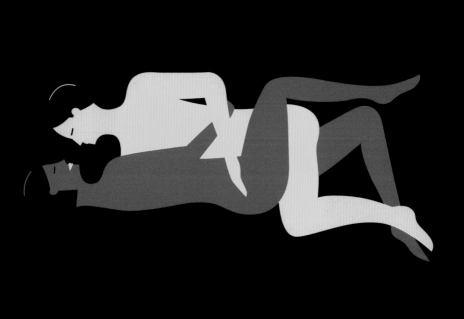

DOGGIE
style ▶▶

There's something very primal about doing the deed from behind that brings out the animal in even the most mild-mannered guy. Plus, doggie positions him for hitting your G-spot—again, and again, and again. Try these moves to amp up your pleasure next time you're going doggie.

BEGINNER

el classico

The classic doggie style is with both of you on your knees. You can get on all fours, but for deeper penetration lay your face all the way down, keeping your **booty** in the air.

INTERMEDIATE

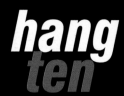

hang ten

While standing up, bend forward with your legs spread slightly, your back straight, and your hands resting on your knees for balance. Your guy enters you from behind, pulling himself as close to you as possible while holding your torso for support. Have him bring you **even closer** until your bodies come into full contact. He leans slightly over you to gain pumping power.

the dragon

Lie on your stomach with your arms raised above your head. With a pillow or two placed under your pubic bone, **spread** your legs slightly. Have your partner stretch his body over yours and enter you, mimicking the position that you're in. Instead of fast from-behind thrusting, this **steamy stance** require a circular, swirling motion.

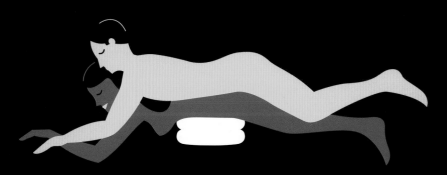

doggie domination

With your guy lying flat on his back, **straddle** his legs on all fours, facing his feet. Keeping your hands on the bed, lower your butt so that he can enter you. This angle is great for a couple of reasons—one, because you're technically on top, thus controlling the pace and depth of penetration. And two, you are in the perfect **G-spot-stimulating** position.

the magic carpet ride

If you don't own a shag rug, then get yourself to Bed Bath & Beyond and throw down $19.99 for a bath mat, pronto. Slip a **vibrator** underneath the mat (this way the sensation isn't too intense), then lie down and position your pelvis over the vibrating area while your guy kneels above you and enters you. He'll have to cobra his back and use a rocking motion—which is ideal, since his movement will help you **grind** against that spot.

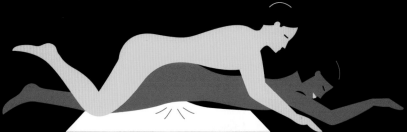

ADVANCED

head over heels

Start by lowering yourself to your knees and crossing your arms on the ground in front of you, using a pillow to cushion your elbows. Stick your butt in the air and rest your head on your arms, **bracing** it on the floor if you need to. Tell your man to stand behind you and lift your legs up by your ankles until your body is almost perpendicular to the floor. Keep your knees bent and have him **enter** you from behind.

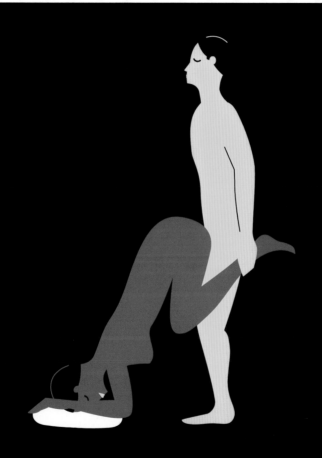

Every time I have doggie-style sex, I experience pain. Is there an angle or technique that will make it feel good?

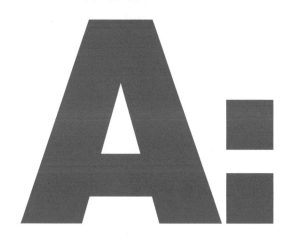

Sex from behind allows the guy to penetrate very deeply inside you, and it might be too deep for your comfort. Instead, lie on your side with him behind you, also on his side. This position allows you to hold his hips and guide him into you, so you can control the depth of his thrusts.

feel good moves for every shape

PENISES CAN TAKE MANY FORMS, and there are perks to almost all of them. Here's how to get maximum satisfaction no matter what he's got going on.

① CURVED TO ONE SIDE: With a slight curve, your guy may hit a sweet spot you never knew you had. Once he's inside you, move your hips from side to side until you find a position that provides a little extra *mmm*.

② CURVED TOWARD HIS NAVEL: This shape is perfect for stimulating your G-spot. Have him get on top of you in a modified missionary position with your legs wrapped around his waist.

③ WIDER THAN IT IS LONG: You-on-top is best for a guy this size since it'll allow him to go as deep as possible. To make him feel even bigger, gyrate in a circular motion, and let him hit every inch of your vaginal walls.

④ LONG AND THIN: Doggie style is great for accommodating a longer guy. The position takes up some of the length, making it extra comfy for you. For more pleasure, contract your PC muscles while he's inside you.

make SOME ▶▶ NOISE!

cording to research,
people who make noise in bed
ave better sex. Try these out
next time you're getting busy. . . .

the *low moan*

Without noise, there's no connection. So give your guy some **verbal signals** right when the action starts. A throaty moan is a good one for showing him that you're into what he's doing so far.

the *sexy sigh*

Maybe your guy hit the perfect spot, then moved on to something else— or a different position entirely. To get him to go back to what he was doing in a positive way, **guide his hand**, body, or face to where he was and give him a sexy sigh to show you loved his previous moves.

the *satisfied* whisper

The way a couple communicates during sex is typically a mirror to how they communicate during a relationship. Try to **open up in bed** as you would with your guy in nonsexual moments to get past any shyness you may feel about giving directions during sex. When you're really feeling it, lean over and whisper, "That feels good," or "Keep doing that" in his ear.

the *happy* grunt

When you're almost there, show him by letting go of your inhibitions and **grunting** with the pace of your thrusts. By being noisy, you'll come across as more sexually confident.

the big finish

If you're not very vocal, it can be hard for a guy to know if you've had an orgasm. A lot of men actually have a tough time reading their partners during sex in general, so noise at the end at least conveys to your partner that you're having a **good time**. Do whatever feels natural here, from a passionate "Oooh yes" to a long, worn-out sigh.

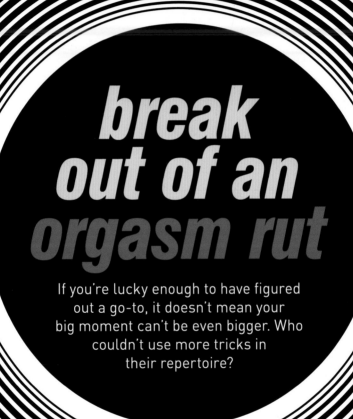

break out of an orgasm rut

If you're lucky enough to have figured out a go-to, it doesn't mean your big moment can't be even bigger. Who couldn't use more tricks in their repertoire?

If Girl-on-Top Does It for You

THIS WILL TOO: Missionary using the Coital Alignment Technique (CAT)

Girl-on-top gets you going because of clitoral stimulation. The CAT delivers similar benefits. Get into missionary position and have him position himself so his pelvis is in-line with yours. Then he should use a figure-eight motion to massage your clitoris with his pelvic bone.

If Oral Does It for You

THIS WILL TOO: A little extra lube

What you're responding to during oral is all the lubrication from his mouth combined with pressure from his tongue. A lot of people underuse lube or think it's only for when a woman feels dry—not the case! Have him touch your clitoris during sex with a lubed-up digit.

If Your Vibrator Does It for You

THIS WILL TOO: You time. A lot of it.

Vibrators are great, but they can potentially desensitize you to any other kind of touch, since they're more powerful than any human. (Not a myth, unfortunately!) Want to wean yourself off one? For the next three months, take a half hour a few times a week to experiment with touching yourself in various ways until you find a new go-to.

MASTERING THE sexth senses

Simply touching during nooky is for basic bitches. Steal these moves to tap all five senses, and enjoy blow-your-mind, next-level sex.

SOUND

From kinky whispers to a sexy secret language,
these tricks will boost "aural" up with "oral"
in your sex-move hall of fame.

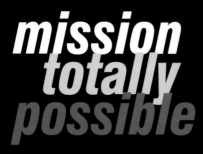

Create a secret couples
code that translates to
sexy-time. Maybe "Order
me a dirty martini" means
"Let's blow this joint . . .
and then each other."

va-va *volume*

Crank up the sound on your next hookup. **Smack his ass** and bang the headboard and let him know you're ready to get wild. Then, entice his D with dirty talk. Tell him—loud and clear—"I love it when you [blank] my [blank]."

beats

Make a playlist to match the beats you want him to hit in bed. Start with something sensual, then go up-tempo so you're both tempted to go Bad Girl Ri Ri during oral.

SIGHT

Guys are visual creatures—this you already know.
(Oh hi, multibillion-dollar porn industry!) But why watch bad
actors have fake sex when you can amp up the visuals
in your own life and both get off?

flash
photography

No man ever got a hard-on looking at a trail of
artfully strewn rose petals. Replace the flowers
with **sexy Polaroids** of yourself in various states
of undress, and leave a trail starting at his door.
Where they lead him is your call, but make sure it's
a spot that's comfortable to roll around in. . . .

ower *show*

Hop in the shower, start soaping up, then holler to your *ovah* to come into the loo. Pull back the shower curtain and **give him a show**—caressing your hair, breasts, hot spot. (If you have a clear shower curtain or glass shower door, all the better.) The sight of your wet-and-wild action should inspire him to hop in and help you reenact those classic Herbal Essences orgasm commercials.

rd's-eye *view*

While riding him, lean way back to give him a **full view** of your sexy self (and increase the depth of penetration). Glance down at him entering you when he's on top. If you're used to hazy, eyes-closed sex, then this will be like Lasik surgery . . . for your vagina.

TASTE

Get a taste of this! No, seriously. Use your tongue in bed in new ways—from sweet to spicy—that will have him drooling.

bone *appetit*

Screw his stomach: The way to a man's heart is through your boobs. **Blindfold him,** dash various sweet treats on your breasts, and lower them into his mouth.

sour *power*

A fun alternative to the old ice-cubes-in-bed trope: **Try frozen grapes** instead. Pop a few in your mouth before a BJ. Lockjaw is a lot easier to deal with when there's a tart, fruity taste involved.

minty fresh

Secretly spread a tiny touch of flavored lube on your lady business. When he goes downtown, the taste will keep him **going for longer**. (Try mint for extra tingles.)

culinary schooled

Christen your kitchen! Push him up against the fridge for a **midcoitus cooldown**, or bend over the counter for easy G-spot access. Then have a snack (postsex pizza, *mmm*).

TOUCH

It's time to get your hands dirty . . . and we mean that in the best possible way.

frisky business

Dress yourself in a **naughty mix** of fabrics that will give him all the feels. Try a lace bra, a silk robe, and velvet undies. Then, hop on top of your man, let him feel the smooth silk stroke his chest, and let the soft velvet graze his package while you straddle him. By the time you get to skin-on-skin, you'll both be hot as hell.

what a stud

Try a studded condom like Durex's Intense Sensations. Tons of tiny, raised dots provide **extra texture and stimulation.**

soft . . . then hard

The touch, the feel of cotton is lovely, but so is a soft, smooth minivibrator on your clitoris. The latest and greatest sex toys are made of luxe, silky silicone that feels soft to the touch. **Pulse a vibe** against the hood of your clit during doggie—or very lightly against your guy's testicles during a BJ. One thing that won't be soft for long? Him.

cold sweats

Head downtown on your guy for a minute, treating him to the natural warmth of your mouth and tongue. Then, change things up and give him a **sensual shock**. Suck on an ice pop, then suck on *his* pop. It'll be cool for him to feel a brand-new temperature mid-action.

SCENT

Olfactory? Try olf*ctory! Researches found
that women rank a guy's scent as their number one turn-on.
Get a whiff of these tips. . . .

eau de orgasm

Spray your sexiest perfume in the air over his workbag—
the strategically placed scent is a stealth way of **planting
naughty thoughts** of you in his head all day.

sexy memory lane

Studies show that scents linked to positive memories
turn women on like mad—especially familiar scents
like barbecue, coffee, clean laundry, and sunblock. So
do a lot of delicates—**then jump his bones**.

phero-*moan*

Stop and smell the . . . sex-sweat? Yes, researchers at Rice University found that pheromones (natural chemicals that attract the opposite sex) emitted by a guy's sweat can **trigger** an emotional response in a woman. So inhale deep, like in yoga, and *namaste*, baby.

rub-a-dub-dub

Try some aphrodisiac bath salts: Lavender and pumpkin pie scents **increase male arousal** up to 40 percent, according to the Smell & Taste Treatment and Research Foundation in Chicago.

KINKY ▶▶
quickies

A recent study found that people who engage in a little kink are happier and more secure in their relationships than the all-vanilla set. If the idea of S&M tickles your pickle, but you don't have the energy to turn your bedroom into a "red room," try these!

① THE QUIET ZONE

Not being "allowed" to make any noise can be a **huge turn-on.** Stuff your thong or his tie into his mouth, then do dirty, dirty things to him until he's digging his nails into his palms to keep from ripping out that gag.

② THE NOONER

Meet him for a mid-workday roll in the hay. First: Raid the supply closet. Snag a ruler (to **spank** him with) and a highlighter (to grade his performance). Be his demanding boss (or vice versa) and scribble an A+ on his inner thigh after he attends to your executive needs.

3 TOOLS OF THE TRADE

If it's going to be **quick and dirty,** be creative with belts, scarves, and tights (just know your tights won't make it back to you in one piece). Use his belt to thwack his butt when he's being bad. Or, let him rip open your tights the second you come home from work, and do it right there against the door, your skirt hiked up against your waist.

TRY SOME INVISIBLE BONDAGE

You don't need tools to bind. Have him command you to hold a position ("put your arms above your head and don't you dare move them"). Or, push his arms behind his back and tell him to keep 'em there—or else. Use your **dirty imaginations** to decide what the consequences are for disobeying.

5 EVOKE HIS BLIND AMBITION

You wake up with two and a half minutes to spare before your alarm rings. Rip off the cami you slept in and tie it over his eyes. Now you can **spin a fantasy** using nothing but your words. Here, we'll get you started: "All the neighbors are crowded around the windows right now, watching us. . . ."

6

THE MULTITASK

There's something really bad about going about your business while your guy *gives* you the business. Call him into the bathroom while you're putting on your makeup, getting ready for a night out. **Lift up** the back of your robe and lean forward, resting your arms against the sink in front of you. Continue to contour your eyes while he enters you from behind. Just know that this is *not* the time to apply liquid eyeliner.

REV YOUR ENGINE

When he takes you out for a fancy occasion, park the car at the most underground point in the garage. Then **straddle him** while he's buckled up (and still at your mercy) and show him *just* how much you appreciate his gesture.

MAKE A
STOPWATCH
SEXY

Not everyone is an orgasm sprinter. (For you long-distancers, a vibrator is a quickie clutch—and speaking of clutch, some are so small, they actually fit in your cute going-out one.) **Challenge** your guy to get you off in record time, and make a deal that if he comes before you do, he's your sex slave for a week. Win-win.

SEX POSITIONS for show-offs

Between the athletic moves, the moans of ecstasy, and the climactic finishes, these gold-medal moves are almost, shall we say, Olympian? (Do try these at home!)

the bawdy bobsled

Two words: *sexual sleigh.* Have your man lie down in bed and slip into reverse cowgirl. Then have him sit up, settle into a **saucy position,** let his hands roam over your breasts and clitoris . . . and enjoy the ride!

the *heavenly* *spiral*

Lie on the bed facedown with your legs hanging off the side while he stands behind you. Then have him enter from behind while he holds your legs at his sides, with **VIP access** to your G-spot.

the long pole

Lie on your back and lift your legs, pressed together, straight up in the air. Then, have your guy kneel in front of you, and put your legs over one of his shoulders as he **leans forward** to hit your G-spot.

oves for
EVERY
MOOD ▶▶

e a woman of many moods, and sometimes those
are not consistent with having insane, contortionist,
over-backward-and-balance-on-your-hand sex.
times, though, that sounds just about right.) Keeping
mind, we've paired amazing sex moves to different
. So go ahead: Get crazy. Or don't!

CUDDLY

When you just wanna snuggle up, lie with your head on his chest and trace cute little messages across his chest ("So happy," "You're hot"). Then let him **reciprocate** by writing his own love note across your back.

NAUGHTY

Go commando on a date. While he's driving or while you're sitting in the movie theater, slyly slip his hand underneath your skirt and give him a saucy little smile. He'll know that when you get home later, it's on like Donkey Kong.

LAZY

Have a pizza picnic party in bed. No TV allowed—
put on a sexy playlist and sit across from each
other like you would at a restaurant. Serve the
pizza on plates, pour some wine, and don't be
afraid to **get messy** with the mozzarella.

 # CRAZY

Doggie-style sex—in front of a window!—taps into
your wild, exhibitionist side. You'll literally **steam
things up.** If you have nosy neighbors, be sure to
do it at night, with the lights off.

SEXY

There are days when you are *on*: Your hair is behaving brilliantly, and you're owning your skinny jeans—and those are the days to **show off the goods.** Straddle him while he's lying on his back, and lean your elbows back so they're resting behind you. Your body should form a semi-bridge. From here, let him do the work. He can thrust up while getting an eyeful of your rocking bod. It's a **total rush** knowing that he's taking in every inch of you and loving it.

6 SHY

Then there are the days when you're not feeling so skinny-jeans ready. . . . This is the perfect time to employ **half-dressed sex:** Keep your minidress on, push your undies aside, and don't let him get totally naked either—it'll feel urgent and charged, without putting you on full display.

STRESSED

Orgasms are tension-busters, so after a hard day at work, pull your guy close and whisper, "All I want is for you to **make me come**." *Hello.* When there's a problem, men like to fix it, so you're making him feel like a total stud while getting yours at the same time.

GROGGY

There's just something about slow, **languid sex** after a late night. Spooning is perfect because 1) it allows you to remain lazily on the bed, and 2) his hands are free to roam your body, meaning even less work for you to do in your sleepy, possibly hungover state. Roll on your side and **guide him** inside you.

VOYEURISTIC

Ask him to **touch himself** while you watch. It's hot to see your guy completely lose control while you maintain it. Plus—learning opportunity!

GENEROUS

'Tis better to give rather than receive, right? "Yes!" says every boyfriend ever. When the **mood strikes**, tell him to lie back and relax, then roll a condom on him and start going down on him. After a few minutes, take it off and continue. Going from sheathed to **bare-skinned** suddenly will make your mouth and tongue feel so much more intense than usual.

11

PLAYFUL

Play-wrestling can be supersexy and fun.
We know it sounds weird, but hear us out:
All that pushing and rubbing up against
each other, *grrrr*. Just be sure to hold the
smackdown on an area with a soft surface—
like your mattress or a fuzzy carpet. There
are no losers in this round. . . .

12 NOSTALGIC

Remember how exciting it was to make out when you were a freshman in high school? Tap into that. Rather than rushing into sex, go for **ten solid minutes** of kissing, groping, and dry humping (grossest term ever, we know, but all the friction it creates is very girl-orgasm friendly)—and that's it. PG-13, highly underrated!

SUBMISSIVE

Tell him to **bind your wrists** behind your back or to your headboard with one of his silk ties before he goes down on you. It's much more comfortable than a pair of handcuffs. (Trust us.)

14 TAKE CHARGE

Climb on top of him and pin his wrists against the bed. Holding on to his arms gives you leverage so you can **really go for it**, and it adds to the you-in-control vibe. The diagonal angle also provides **more contact** between his pelvic bone and your clitoris, upping the orgasmic potential.

15 KINKY

On nights when you want to let your freak flag fly, assume an **alter ego**. (What? Beyoncé does it! Sasha Fierce, anyone?) It's easier to get into character when you don't look like you, so meet him at the door wearing a wig. Tell him that "Erin is working late. I'm her evil twin." His night just got a *lot* more interesting.

16 PATIENT

When you want to draw out the experience, try **stop-and-go sex**. How it works: Bring yourselves to the brink, then stop. Don't move, don't grind, don't do anything for at least thirty seconds. Then resume your activities, and repeat the stop-and-go at least two more times. Delaying the release will make your orgasm feel superhuman **powerful**.

17 EXPERIMENTAL

Hot-and-cold play is not Chris Martin's experimental side band: It's when you alternate the sensations to **build tension**, because you don't know what you're going to get next. Take turns blindfolding each other and teasing sensitive spots, like the neck, nipples, and inner thighs, with ice cubes and your **warm breath**.

18 ROMANTIC

Dim lighting plus backrub equals *très* romantic, and a massage candle kills two lovebirds (Thank you, we'll be here all week) with one stone. Babeland sells one that melts into a shea butter–infused oil. A **massage** also releases the bonding hormone oxytocin, so you'll feel even more connected to each other postrub.

five moves

for THREE

MORE ▶▶

MOODS

A new study proves you can up your odds of climaxing by trying five different moves during sex. Get ready to rack up the Os.

FIVE MOVES FOR WHEN YOU WANT TO TAKE CHARGE

1 Have him lie on the bed, then stand up and invite him to watch while you softly stroke yourself all over.

----

2 Step closer to the mattress, take his hand, and guide it between your legs. Let him see the pleasure register on your face as he stimulates your clitoris.

----

3 Climb on top of the bed so you're hovering over him on all fours, with your legs on either side of his torso and your breasts at his face level. Alternate dipping each of your nipples into his mouth.

----

4 Flip around, and go down on him with your head facing his feet and your backside and girl bits on eye-popping display.

----

5 Transition into cowgirl position, and touch yourself as you grind against him in slow, erotic circles.

FIVE MOVES FOR WHEN YOU CRAVE A QUICKIE

1 Sit him down, and straddle just one of his legs. As you make out, rub your clitoris against his thigh to get yourself going.

---

2 Take his penis in your mouth and go all the way down on him (or as far as you can). The suddenness will rev him from 0 to 50.

---

3 Now that his penis is lubed up with your saliva, use it as a sex toy by pressing it against your clitoris and sliding it back and forth.

---

4 Get into doggie position, and then take his hand and press it against your clitoris with your hand on top to ensure you get the exact pressure/movement you need.

---

5 Finish things off by moving your legs closer together—the extratight fit will make things more intense, pushing you both over the edge.

FIVE LIE-BACK-AND-ENJOY MOVES

1 Rub his scalp mid-kiss. Press in the pads of your fingers, and slowly drag them to the top of his neck.

----

2 Place his hands on your waist, fingers up, and have him slide his palms up and down, teasingly grazing the sides of your boobs.

----

3 Next, move his hands to your inner thighs. Have him tease you so that he comes thisclose to your clitoris.

----

4 Start giving him oral, and while you do, massage his butt, making your way to his perineum (between his butt and balls). Use two fingers to rub in a circular motion.

----

5 When he finishes, have him go down on you while stroking your pubic area just outside your labia. He should also use his fingers on your C-spot while he kisses the area around it.

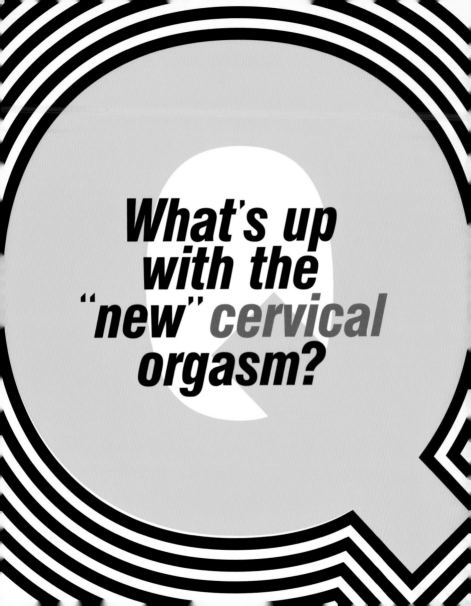

What's up with the "new" cervical orgasm?

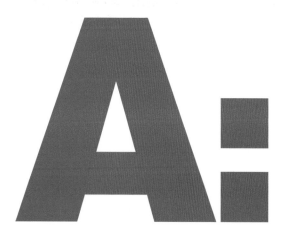

Consider the cervix—the one-inch area connecting the top of your vagina to your uterus—the new frontier in orgasms. Sometimes called full-body orgasms, cervical Os are different from clitoral and G-spot varieties we know and love, because the cervix is deeper in the body, rarely touched, and highly sensitive—stimulating it can potentially radiate pleasure throughout the body. Discover a cervical O with a G-spot vibrator or a fantastic penis, long enough to press against the cervix. Get aroused first—increased blood flow through your happy place will make the cervix easier to access. Then try slow circles, like you're giving your cervix a massage. You'll know it's the C-spot when your entire body tingles in ecstasy.

TROUBLESHOOTING:
how to
help
him help
you

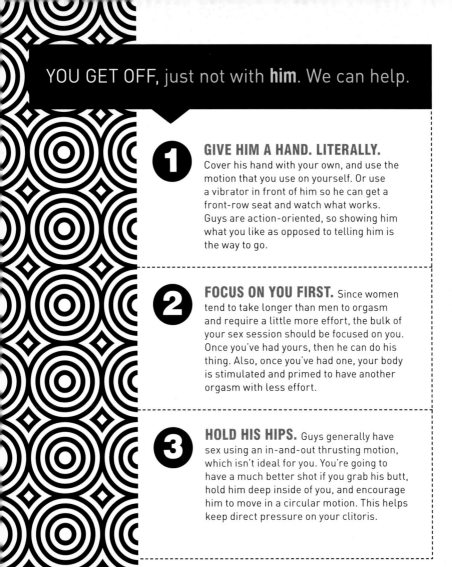

YOU GET OFF, just not with **him**. We can help.

1 GIVE HIM A HAND. LITERALLY.

Cover his hand with your own, and use the motion that you use on yourself. Or use a vibrator in front of him so he can get a front-row seat and watch what works. Guys are action-oriented, so showing him what you like as opposed to telling him is the way to go.

2 FOCUS ON YOU FIRST.

Since women tend to take longer than men to orgasm and require a little more effort, the bulk of your sex session should be focused on you. Once you've had yours, then he can do his thing. Also, once you've had one, your body is stimulated and primed to have another orgasm with less effort.

3 HOLD HIS HIPS.

Guys generally have sex using an in-and-out thrusting motion, which isn't ideal for you. You're going to have a much better shot if you grab his butt, hold him deep inside of you, and encourage him to move in a circular motion. This helps keep direct pressure on your clitoris.

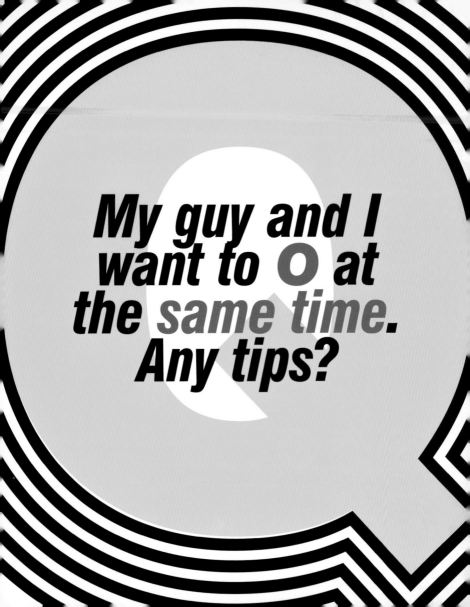

A:

Because orgasming from intercourse alone is tough for a solid 70 percent of women, according to studies, go for situations that *you* find most orgasmic. Into deep penetration? Try positions like the Speed Bump that tickle the G-spot, suggests Tiffanie Henry, PhD, a sex therapist in Atlanta. "You lie flat on your tummy with a pillow under your pelvis, then spread 'em as he enters from the rear," she says. If clitoral stimulation is your jam, massage your pleasure button as you're doing it. The classic 69 position is always an oral option for synchronized O'ing. Henry also suggests tantric yoga with your partner—intimate couples poses and breathing exercises can help you "achieve orgasm with rhythmic precision."

233

PART 3

advanced
techniques

all right, so you know how to do it in missionary,

you know how to rock it in doggie, and you're looking for something a little more . . . **outré.** Are you interested in threesomes? A little kink? A little **backdoor booty?** Or maybe just some sex positions that look like they might require advanced yoga training and a heck of a lot of practice to pull off? Whatever it is your wanton little **heart desires,** we've got it covered in this chapter. So go ahead: **Experiment.**

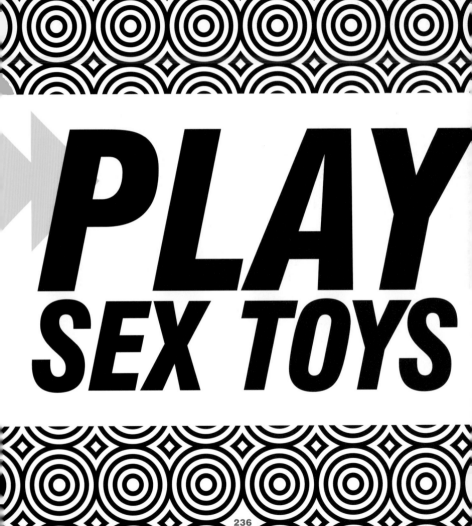

PLAY
SEX TOYS

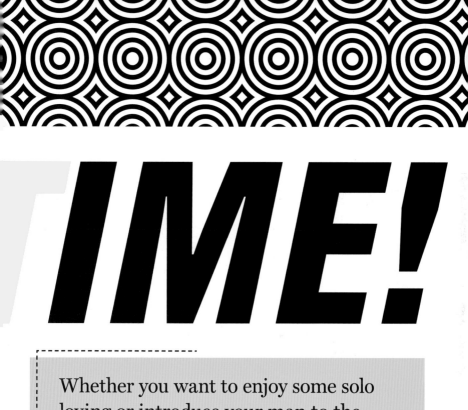

TIME!

Whether you want to enjoy some solo loving or introduce your man to the **EXPLOSIVE** pleasure your vibrator can bring, our guide to **SEX TOYS** ensures you'll never run out of sexy tricks and tips.

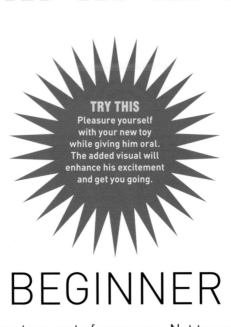

TRY THIS
Pleasure yourself with your new toy while giving him oral. The added visual will enhance his excitement and get you going.

BEGINNER

So sex toys sort of scare you. Not to worry: Introducing a motorized device to your delicate flower can be a downright delightful experience. Try a bullet, or something equally small for a sweet experience for beginners. Try: **a** Babeland™ Silver Bullet ($15), **b** Fun Factory™ UFO ($100), **c** Jimmyjane Little Chroma™ ($125)

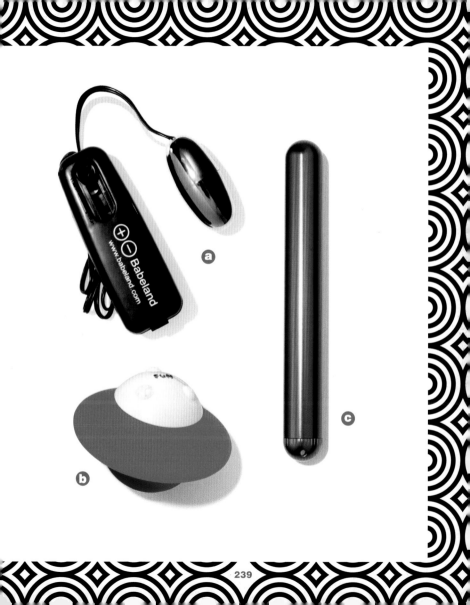

INTERMEDIATE

You're beyond bullets but not quite ready for butt plugs. Welcome to the intermediate playfield of XXX-level shopping: naughty pieces that offer the potential for double orgasms. Try: 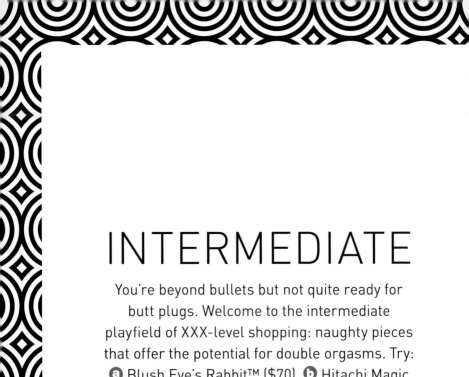 Blush Eve's Rabbit™ ($70), Hitachi Magic Wand™ ($55), Je Joue™ Mio cock ring ($109)

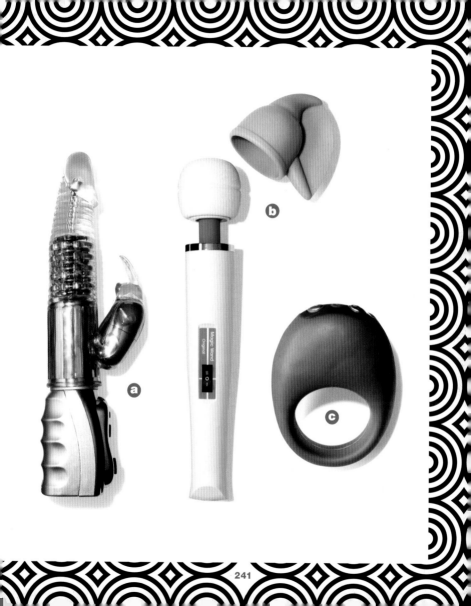

ADVANCED

A master of sex toys, you're so advanced, you could school Christian Grey in kinky crop-spanking. Try: ⓐ Ohmibod® Lovelife Adventure Triple Stim Vibrator ($99), ⓑ Lelo Luna Beads™ ($47), ⓒ Sportsheets® Studded XO Crop ($17)

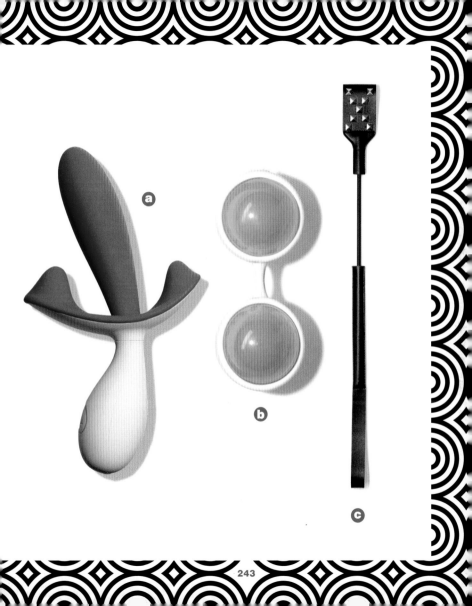

how to get your GUY TO LOVE ▶▶ SEX TOYS

Guys are sometimes weirded out by sex toys in the bedroom. If your partner recoils when you bust ou toy, use these tips to get him comfortable with it g Think of it as slowly going down the stairs in a too pool, except in this case, the pool is full of dildos.

① START SMALL, LITERALLY

Smaller, **less intimidating** vibrators are a good start. "I tend to advise starting with a toy that's more couples-related," says sex and relationships author Ian Kerner. "That's a good way of making it about the two of you as opposed to a large pink fake penis." Even giving the sex toy to your partner so that he's the one controlling it (and, subsequently, your pleasure) can make him feel better about having something new in the bedroom.

2 GO FOR NOVELTY

Handcuffs, sex chairs, lubricants, and role-playing are all kinky good ways to **change up** your normal sex routine.

3 GO SHOPPING TOGETHER

Just go to a store and look. If the idea of ducking into your local sex-toy dealer seems shady, you can just **browse online**.

4 DON'T BE AFRAID TO LAUGH

The key is for both of you to remember that sex should be fun. You're bringing your **favorite toys** out, and you're both making it work with each other, except instead of G.I. Joes and Barbies, it's Rabbit vibrators and sex cushions. Or maybe it is G.I. Joes and Barbies. No judgment.

toys ▶▶ for HIM

Rolling up to bed with a giant phallic sex toy that's bigger than he is can give him a complex. Instead, try the Je Joue Mim ($89), an egg-shaped vibrator that fits in the palm of your hand. **Pulse it** on your clitoris during doggie or against his perineum for a little extra love during oral.

Or, slip the Lovehoney Bionic Bullet Rabbit Vibrating Cock Ring ($23) on his member. It will make him last longer and give you extra pleasure for an increased chance of mutual climax. Everybody wins!

MOVES FOR USING YOUR VIBRATOR ON HIM . . .

A recent Trojan study found that 47 percent of men are open to using a vibrator in bed. Roll your vibe **teasingly** between his thighs, and the vibrations will awaken the nerve endings throughout his entire pelvic region. Add some water-based lube to the vibe, and sweep the tip of your toy back and forth over his frenulum (remember: it's that notch on the underside of his penis where his head and shaft meet). During sex, you can also press it into the back of his perineum, the spot between his balls and his back door—but make sure he's cool with it first! Pulsing against this point **stimulates** his sensitive prostate. Now spread those good vibes!

calling all sex-toy shoppers!

You researched the shit out of your new cell phone before you bought it, so shouldn't you be equally informed about the GADGETS that bring you to orgasm? Embrace these tips like a lover.

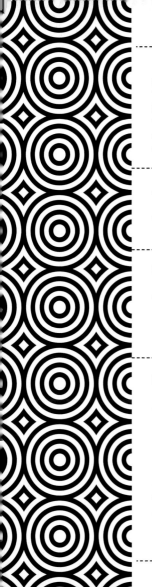

SILICONE IS SEXY . . .
Toys made of this medical-grade material are safest because they're slick—there are no tiny holes that can trap bacteria between sexual adventures. Also saucy and sanitary: glass, stainless steel, and hard plastic get-you-off objects.

. . . PHTHALATES AREN'T
Look for labels announcing toys that are free of these chemicals, which are used to soften everyday plastics but don't necessarily belong inside your vagina.

PLAY GREEN
If you want to make Mother Nature as happy as you will be, look for the new wave of sexessories with rechargable, cell-like batteries that power up via USB port. These snazzy toys are often pricier, but they also buzz harder and last longer. . . .

BAWDY BUYER, BEWARE
Make sure you're not paying for a used sex toy (gag) by shopping at a toy boutique whose policy is to accept returns for broken playthings. Also note privacy policies: If you don't want your mailman or roommate to know you've bought a vibe, order online from the best in the naughty business, like Babeland or the Pleasure Chest. Both use covert names that won't embarrass you on your credit card statement and plain shipping boxes with no store logo. Business on the outside, sex party on the inside!

GET YOUR
SEX TOYS
squeaky-
CLEAN ▶▶

Soft rubber or jelly-based sex toys often carry HPV even after they're washed, according to an Indiana University study. The solution: Choose vibrators and other toys made of the materials below. After removing the batteries (and warning your roommate), clean them after each use in these ways:

MATERIAL	HOW TO CLEAN
GLASS	Like fragile wineglasses, most glass sex toys don't handle hot temps well. Wash with warm water and soap only.
LEATHER	Wipe it down with rubbing alcohol.
SILICONE	Wash with unscented dish soap and warm water, and air-dry. Or place in the top rack of a dishwasher.
SOFT VINYL/HARD PLASTIC	Plastic is more porous than silicone and so more susceptible to HPV. Wipe carefully with a cloth dipped in warm, soapy water.
STAINLESS STEEL	Immerse in boiling water for ten minutes.

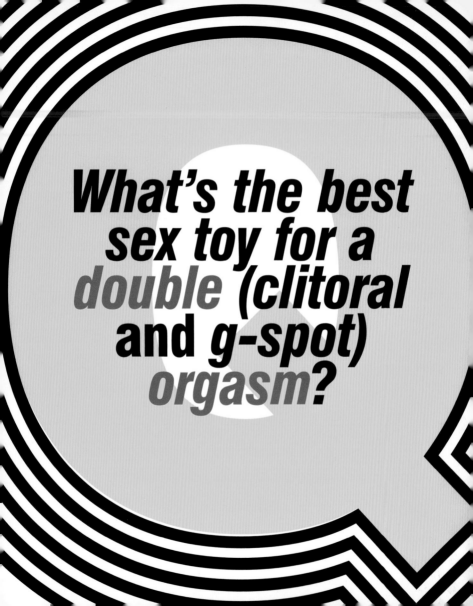

What's the best sex toy for a double (clitoral and g-spot) orgasm?

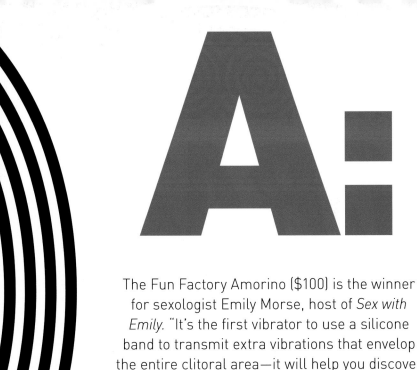

The Fun Factory Amorino ($100) is the winner for sexologist Emily Morse, host of *Sex with Emily.* "It's the first vibrator to use a silicone band to transmit extra vibrations that envelop the entire clitoral area—it will help you discover nerve endings you didn't even know you had." Plus, the tip is perfect for G-spot stimulation— it's upturned toward the sexual heavens.

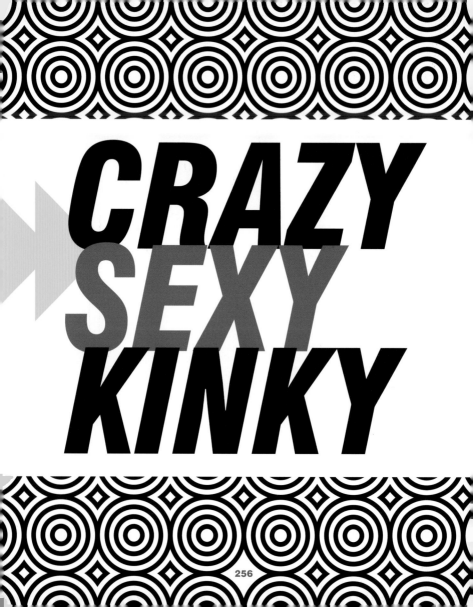

CRAZY
SEXY
KINKY

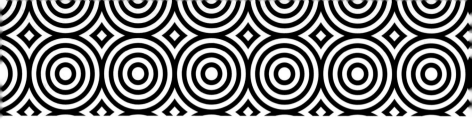

A recent study found that couples who engage in a little KINK are happier in their relationships.

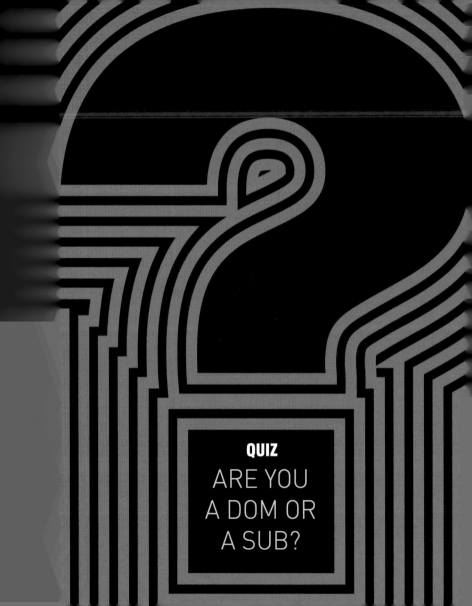

QUIZ

ARE YOU
A DOM OR
A SUB?

Find out if you're a Christian or an Ana in bed.

You order kale at your favorite restaurant. The waiter brings you spinach instead. You:

a. Meekly eat the inferior greens.

b. Demand to speak to the manager and leave with a lifetime of comped meals.

You discovered an anonymous coworker took your stapler. Your response is to:

a. Buy another stapler and write "For Everyone to Use <3" on it in glitter.

b. Send an all-company e-mail with the subject line "TO WHATEVER PIECE OF HUMAN SCUM TOOK MY STAPLER."

You're looking for a partner who knows:

a. The knots you prefer to be tied up with.

b. His place. (Hint: It's on his knees.)

MOSTLY As: SUB

Submitting to someone else is your strongest aphrodisiac. The fact that you're willing to let go and indulge your darkest fantasies is pretty baller.

MOSTLY Bs: DOM

You get off on your partner submitting to your whims, from whips and chains to dirty talk that would make E. L. James blush.

P.S. Some people go both ways. They're called switches.

three
secret
KINK PROPS
hiding in
YOUR HOUS

1. HAIR ELASTIC = HANDCUFFS

Use it to bind his wrists.

2. HAIRBRUSH = PADDLE

Volumizing boar bristles feel naughty on a bare bum.

3. ELECTRIC TOOTHBRUSH = VIBRATOR

Hold the base against your clitoris during sex.

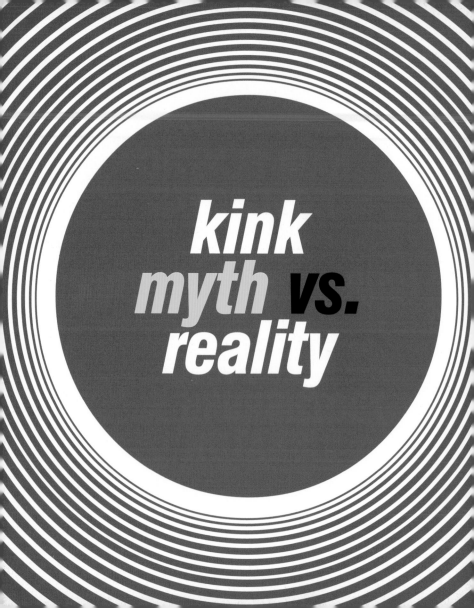

kink
myth **vs.**
reality

Myth: Kink is all about pain.

Reality: It's all about taking control of or giving control to your partner . . . and maybe some pain that you happen to find hot or pleasurable.

Myth: Only sexual deviants with broken pasts are into BDSM.

Reality: It's a perfectly healthy sexual flavor, not unlike, say, shower sex.

Myth: A woman who's submissive isn't a feminist.

Reality: If being a sub turns you on and you're asking for exactly that, you're a feminist.

EGINNER
KINK ▸▸

Baby steps! Try kink on for size with these sexy (not scary) moves.

1 PEEK-A-BOOB
Kink 101: Dress the part with see-through lingerie. Sheer laciness surrounding your body will make you feel like a sensual superstar.

----

2 MY TIES
The LBD of BDSM: versatile ties that can be worn as a blindfold as a painless way to tie your (or his) wrists above your (or his) head. When you can't see or use your hands, all you can focus on is *Holy sh*t, where will his fingers go next?*

----

3 THE ART OF THE TICKLE
Use a feather tickler to dust off your bookshelf—or to tickle your man's nips (and other tender parts). Don't knock it till you try it: Feather-on-skin is a highly underrated tingly turn-on.

----

4 KINKY BOOTS
Stage your own off-off-Broadway production, starring you in the role of "irresistible dominatrix" and costarring your boyfriend in the role of "guy who's been very, very bad."

INTERMEDIATE
KINK ▶▶

You've mastered the basic bitch moves of kink. Now here's how to up your game.

PRETTY IN KINK
Tie yourself up in racy ribbons that would make Martha Stewart shudder. A cupless bra and crotchless panty (the French call them *ouverts*) have never looked so lovely. . . .

CUFF LOVE
Loop a pair of cuffs around a bedpost or bannister, and have him bind your hands before he gives you the goods.

DON'T RULE IT OUT
A ruler is excellent when paired with role-play, like a professor catching his student texting under the table.

DVANCED
KINK ▶▶

Let's just say this isn't your first rodeo. You're ready for a flogger and you don't care who knows it. Keep your routine fresh with a few new tricks. . . .

BEN WA
Get some Ben Wa balls and keep them in you, whether you're having sex or just casually walking down the street. So ballsy . . .

PINCH PLEASURE
Ask him to slip on some nipple clamps at the widest angle of the clamp for the least pain. When you take them off, the blood rushes to your girls.

SCARY-SEXY
A Wartenberg wheel may look like a ravioli cutter, but when your partner runs it over your inner thigh, its tickling touch will have you begging for more.

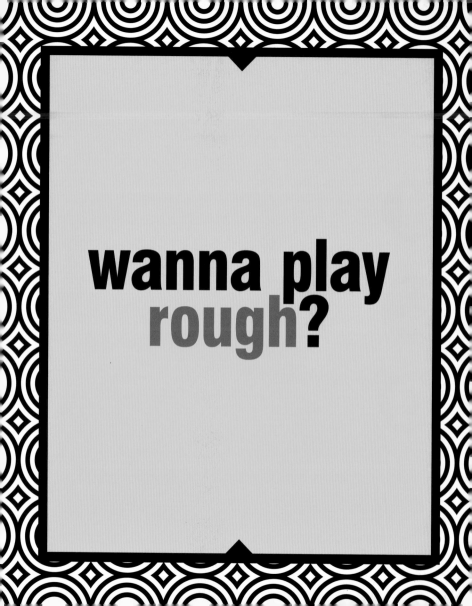

YOU KNOW HOW IT'S EASIER to jump into a cold swimming pool and get it over with, rather than slowly wade in? The exact opposite is true of rough sex. Here's how to test the waters.

1 START SMALL, AND GO SLOWLY

Establish what's okay and what's not before even starting (aka force is cool, name-calling isn't). Test out some light spanking, getting held down, etc. Then if you're both comfortable and turned on, keep going. . . .

2 RAMP UP THE INTENSITY

Try using restraints, or slightly harder hitting, or having your partner put a hand on your neck and gently (gently!) tilt it up. Always have a safe word at the ready (when you say *pinkie*, that means a hard stop), and make the dominant partner ask for what he wants. "Can I spank you?" "Yes, please spank me."

3 SWITCH IT UP, IN TERMS OF WHO'S DOMINANT

That way you can both experience what it's like to be in control . . . and what it's like to give it up.

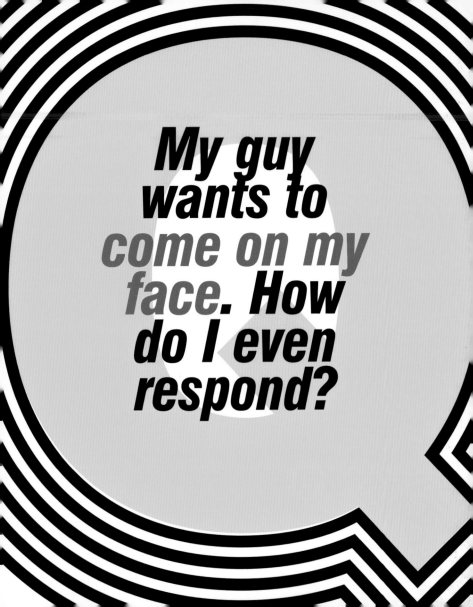

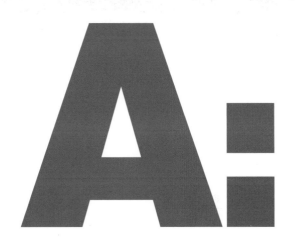

A:

If you're down to do this, go for it. But if you're not so enthused, ask why he wants to. That way, you're at least *trying* to get his logic . . . always a good thing. If he says it's hot, suggest he come on your chest (still hot, not so skeevy). If he's into dominating, try doctor/patient role-play. But don't feel pressured into a "face job." It's extreme.

FIFTY
SHADES
of SEX ▶▶

It's no wonder *Fifty Shades of Grey* sold a gazillion copies: Anastasia Steele and Christian Grey have some hot sex. We'll show you how to re-create their steamiest moves, but fair warning: These are not for the faint of heart. Get ready to step into the red room. . . .

the anastasia
demand

From behind, have him **thrust deeply** into you at an extremely slow pace. After several thrusts, he should pull back and wait until you demand he continue. Thrusting should then recommence.

the beltway

Have him tie you up, blindfold you, and drag a belt from your stomach to your clitoris, **stimulating** you there until you come.

ben wa
xperience

Bend over, grab your ankles, and have your man **nsert** Ben Wa balls into your vagina. Walk around or get into water, like Anastasia did) with the balls inside of you. Then lie across his lap with your butt facing up. He should **rub** your butt, moving from your cheeks down to your clitoris. The balls inside you, along with his touch, will create an intense sensation.

the
bedpost
bend

While tied to the bedposts and lying on your stomach, lift your butt up and have him enter you from behind. Grip the bedpost tightly and **push back** against him.

fifty shades of flogging

Have your man tie you up and blindfold you. Put on headphones. Have him **cuff** your arms and legs to the bed. Start playing music as he lightly slaps your breasts with a flogger. *Then* have him kiss down your body and start performing oral sex. When you're about to **climax**, have him remove your ankle restraints as he lifts you up so your back is arched and only your shoulders are on the bed. He should then thrust into you very slowly, gradually increasing his pace.

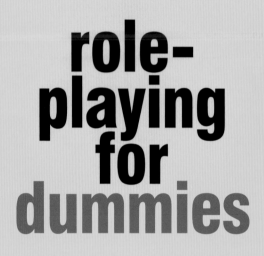

role-playing for dummies

Playing MAKE-BELIEVE
in the bedroom isn't just for
experienced kinksters.

1 **Figure out your fantasy.** Many scenarios—naughty housekeeper, hot professor—sound cliché, but that's because they work! Or maybe you were a lifeguard as a teenager and always wanted to give that cute swimmer mouth-to-mouth. . . .

2 **Now share it.** Bring up your fantasy as a compliment. Say, "I had this really hot dream about you last night. I was a professor and you were my student. . . ." By including your partner from the get-go, you make it clear that your fantasy is just that.

3 **Establish some limits.** Before losing yourself in a character, be sure to let your partner know what you're comfortable doing and what's going too far.

4 **Set the scene.** A wardrobe change isn't mandatory for role-play, but it can definitely be fun. The same goes for dressing up your environment. You probably won't be able to transform your bedroom into a classroom, but wheeling in a chalkboard or a desk can go a long way.

5 **Don't forget to have fun.** Don't get caught up in the theatrics of it all—the aim is to have fun, not win an Oscar. If you break character and burst into laughter, don't sweat it.

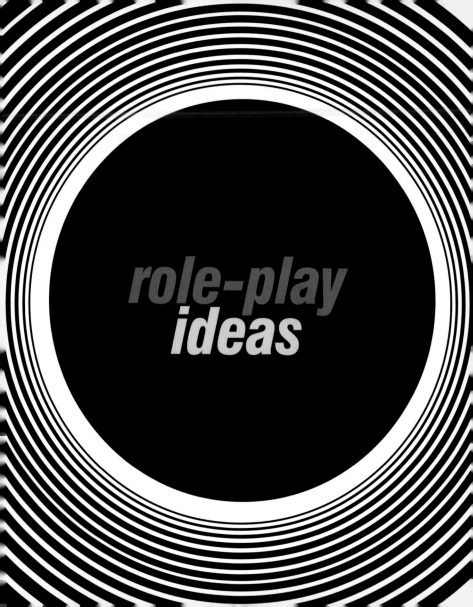

role-play
ideas

1 Watch a sexy movie together, and then act out one of the steamiest scenes as the characters in the film. Already having the visual of who you want to become and what you're going to do to each other can increase the anticipation and ultimately your arousal. *Silver Linings Playbook* is a good recent film, or download *Secretary* for a kinkier option.

2 If you're in a committed relationship, occasionally pretending you're casual f*ck buddies lends sex an edgy feel. You can screw the romance and tenderness for now, and just get dirty.

3 This may sound wacky, but go at it like you're animals—for example, a lion and lioness out in the savannah. It can help you let loose of inhibitions and get ultrawicked between the sheets.

4 There's truth to the phrase "Absence makes the heart grow stronger." When there's an obstacle to reaching your significant other, it heightens erotic tension. So even if you live together, role-play that you're in a long-distance relationship: Head to different rooms and have urgent Skype sex.

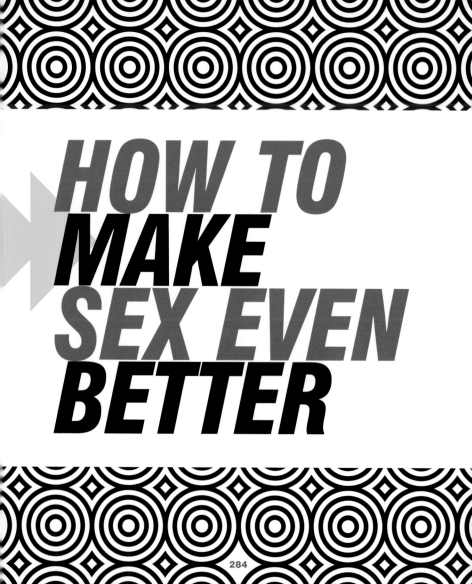

HOW TO MAKE SEX EVEN BETTER

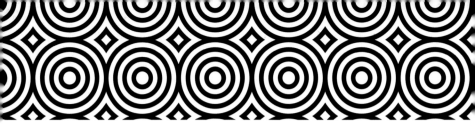

Looking for easy **UPGRADES** to your (let's face it, already pretty great) sex life? Look no further. . . .

EXPERIMENT WITH EDGING

It may sound like something only cool kids do ("Bro, do you even edge?"), but it's really just a way to describe the act of stopping sex right before the point of orgasm to **cool off** a bit before starting up again. Forcing each other to hold off from orgasm can make the eventual release much more intense (and also make him last longer).

ADD A PILLOW IN THERE

No, don't have sex with the pillow; that's weird. But a pillow can modify most positions by slightly altering the angle of penetration, and that can make a **huge difference**.

WEAR
      YOUR
SOCKS

Research shows that keeping your socks
on during sex can help regulate your body
temperature, which in turn makes you
more comfortable and it makes it easier to
orgasm. Keep a pair of socks around *just*
for sex. Sex socks. Sox.

USE A TIE

Modify a position by tying your hands behind your back, above your head, or to the bed. Or use the tie as a **blindfold**. Limiting mobility or covering your eyes and giving control to your partner can make an old position feel totally new. It's like the espresso shot of sex modifiers.

KISS WHILE YOU COME

Kissing during an orgasm adds an emotional intensity, like you can almost feel your partner's orgasm **vibrating** through you.

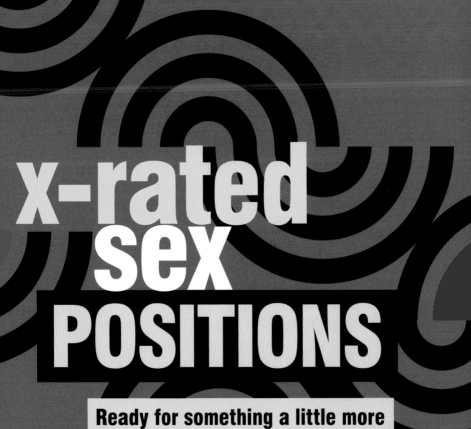

x-rated
sex
POSITIONS

Ready for something a little more raunchy? Beware: The following sex positions are not for shrinking violets.

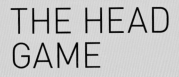

THE HEAD GAME

Start this inverted delight by **lying** flat on the ground faceup. With your hands supporting your lower back, lift your legs and backside way, way up so they're as perpendicular to the ground as you can get them. Have your man kneel before you, **grab your ankles,** and bring his knees to your shoulders. Then take his hands and ask him to hold your hips—that will steady you both. Hold his thighs for leverage and adjust so your genitals can join for some **otherworldly** upside-down action.

THE SOFA SPREAD

Stand on the edge of a couch, a bed, or two chairs with your legs spread wide. Position your man so he's standing on the floor facing you. Adjust the width of your stance (bending your knees slightly if necessary) so he can **easily slide** between them and get your pelvises to meet— then rock your bodies together to feel the **bliss**.

X-RATED

This position is all about control—so take it from the get-go and have your man lie faceup on the bed. Turn around and **straddle** him—so your back is toward him—and then lower yourself onto his erect penis. **Extend** your legs back toward his shoulders, relaxing your torso onto the bed between his feet. With both your legs and your man's forming an X-shape, start to **slide** up and down. Use his feet for added thrusting leverage.

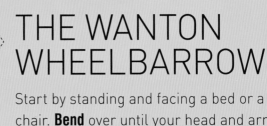

THE WANTON WHEELBARROW

Start by standing and facing a bed or a chair. **Bend** over until your head and arms are resting on its surface. Have your man stand behind you and **grab** one of your ankles. Make sure to keep your knee slightly bent as you shift your weight to the leg that's still on the ground. Lifting your foot to rest near his hip, he should **enter** you from behind.

how to have multiple Os

Women's bodies are hardwired to have more than one feel-good EXPLOSION. Well, hallelujah! Here, we break down how to achieve that ultimate pleasure.

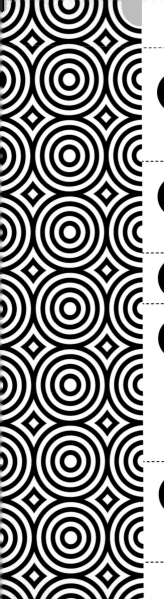

1 Get into the right frame of mind. After you've gotten there for the first time, rather than switching off mentally and sexually—which is what you do when you assume you've reached the finale—you need to remain expectant and open to further arousal.

2 Step up the sexercises. Consider this your ultimate down-there workout motivator: Strong PC muscles have been demonstrated to be a crucial component to having multiples.

3 Max out foreplay. If you're aroused slowly, then you'll stay aroused for longer.

4 Take a mini time out. Once you come for the first time, you're probably in the habit of pulling away from him because you're so sensitive to his touch. But here's the difference between a sack session that finishes with a happy ending and one that continues on to multiple peaks: If you fall into a stupefied pleasure coma, you're done. If you resume touching an area that is not hypersensitive, you bring it on.

5 Keep your position. The key to climaxing is steady stimulation, so when you're almost there, hold off on the erotic acrobatics. Instead, stick with a position that's hitting your hot spots and stay there until you come.

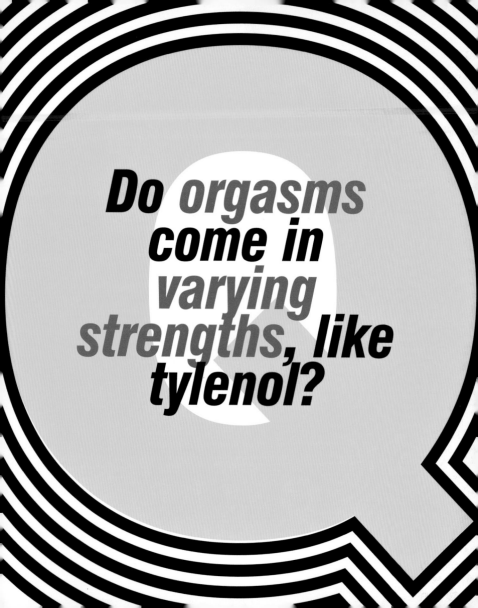

Do orgasms come in varying strengths, like tylenol?

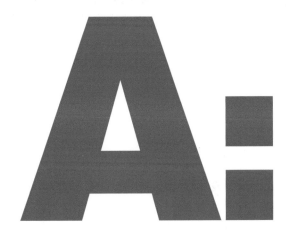
A:

Yes, some women's vaginas are more sensitive and can have stronger orgasms—kinda like your freaky-awesome friend whose boobs you want to steal 'cause she can orgasm from nip action alone. It's a much-repeated tip, we know, but if you're looking for more earth-altering orgasms, every expert recommends Kegel exercises! Regularly flexing those muscles, which run from the inside of your vagina to your lower spine, can make them contract more fiercely during orgasm.

OUTSIDE ▶▶
the bedroom

Sometimes, you don't have the luxury of being in a private bedroom when the mood for sex strikes. And sometimes, getting it on a little more . . . publicly . . . is just what you need to kick your sex life up a notch. Read on for tips on how to do it, wherever you are. . . .

BEFORE
YOU START . . .

1 **Pack the essentials.** Have a sex kit that includes everything from a tarp to lube and even first-aid supplies. Items like candles and a wine bottle opener could come in handy too. If the kit is ready ahead of time, nothing will stand in the way of a spontaneous outdoor tryst.

----

2 **Be aware of your surroundings.** It's not the sexiest thing to think about, but you do need to be aware of your environment while getting busy outside. Look out for critters—like bears, ticks, and ants—that can be attracted to the pheromones given off by humans during sexual activity.

3 **Dress for success.** Wear clothes and shoes that can easily be taken off and on with easy access (think skirts, sandals). Going commando wouldn't hurt, either.

----

4 **Beware bug bites.** Consider mosquito netting that can easily be draped over your bodies and hung on a tree branch. This is a lot sexier than the scent of mosquito repellent on your skin.

----

5 **Stay out of trouble.** Outdoor areas may also be public areas, so map out visibility ahead of time to avoid the embarrassment of being seen.

IN THE GREAT OUTDOORS . . .

pop-a-Squat

Have your partner lie on the ground (in a bed of grass, obviously) and, facing away from him, straddle him and sit down, **reverse-cowgirl** style. You can use a nearby tree stump for support if you need it.

the *blair witch* project

In a dark tent, lie down and point a flashlight at different parts of your body. Your partner has to follow the light, **licking and kissing** everything he sees. This foreplay could get so steamy you'll have to unzip the vent flap.

on a picnic table

First, be sure to check for rusty hardware, ants, and dry rot. All clear? Sit on the edge of the table with your legs on the bench, and have your guy sit on the bench between them, facing you, his head level with **your thighs**. Get it? It's a picnic! And you're so much better than PB&J.

in the ocean

Wade into deep water, and have him stand behind you so that when you start going at it, no one on the beach can tell what you're doing. It'll feel **scandalous** and exciting!

IN A CAR . . .

RULES OF THE ROAD

1 Before you hook up in your car, a newsflash from the fun police: Safe sex means not crashing the car during road head or getting slapped with a public-indecency fine. So before we get started, keep these guidelines in mind, m'kay?

----

2 Park the car and turn it off—nothing says buzzkill like the airbag exploding on your groin.

3 Do it at sunset or later—you'll be less likely to be seen, plus it's cooler out.

----

4 Find a private, kid-free place (along the beach, on a quiet side street, a movie parking lot, even your garage).

----

5 Put a towel or sweatshirt over the seat so 1) your butt doesn't stick to the leather, and 2) you won't have to get your car detailed the next day.

sunny-side *up*

Open the sunroof and have your man sit in the passenger seat. **Climb on top**, facing him, and stand with your feet on either side of his hips (thanks to the sunroof, your upper body will be outside). Let him to treat you to oral—and if you're wearing a skirt or dress, just ditch your underwear and let the material cascade over his head.

take *him* for a ride

With your guy in the passenger seat, shift the seat all the way back, and recline the seat back. Get into his lap and go at it **cowgirl-style**. (Hint: Grab onto the headrest for leverage.)

fast and furious

Kneel on the passenger seat, facing the back of the car, and (depending on how tall he is) have him either kneel on the seat or crouch behind you for doggie sex.

spoonful of
hotness

Spoon sex is the most comfortable backseat option (missionary can feel claustrophobic)—plus, no one will be able to see you. Move the front seats forward and the seat backs upright. He should lie on his side across the backseat, with you in front of him so your back is pressed against his chest. If the seat is narrow, keep yourself from falling off by bracing your hands against the seat in front of you.

IN A POOL . . .

ladder *lovin'*

This position requires some maneuvering. Climb
down to the second-to-last rung of the pool
ladder. Do a 180, holding the rails, so your back is
to the wall. **Lean** forward and spread your legs so
your guy can lower himself behind you and place
his feet between your legs on the rung below you.
Adjust your bodies so he can slip himself inside
you. In this half-in, half-out-of-the-water position,
only your lower bodies are submerged. So each
time your man thrusts, cold water will splash
against your exposed skin, **electrifying** all your
nerve endings.

submarine

Have your man sit on the second or third stair in the shallow end of the pool. **Straddle** his lap and take him inside you. Next, lift your legs so your feet are propped up on the top of the stairs. Have him grab on to your thighs as you lean back. Hold on to his calves to help you stay elevated as he pulls you back and forth. The feeling of weightlessness combined with the sensual deprivation of not being able to hear since your ears are submerged will allow you to surrender to the **bliss** of your partner's member throbbing inside you.

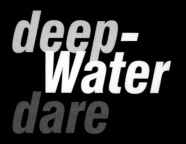

deep-Water dare

When you and your guy are swimming, make your way to chest-high water and stand face-to-face. Hold on to his shoulders as you jump up and **wrap your legs** tightly around his thighs. Have him cradle your butt with both hands to keep you propped up as he enters you. The water will make you weightless so you can easily **glide** back and forth.

tawdry tube

Have your guy sit in an inner tube with his legs dangling over the edge. Then **straddle** his lap while facing him, and slowly lower yourself onto his penis with your hands on his shoulders or the tube for support. Once he's inside you, begin to **rock** back and forth. He can intensify the action by grasping your hips to help propel you.

IN A HOT TUB . . .

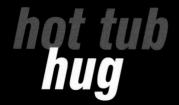

hot tub
hug

Start with your guy sitting on the bench with his knees bent and legs slightly spread, leaning back with his arms outstretched and resting on the edge of the tub. Straddle him, facing forward, and **lower yourself** onto his penis, holding on to his shoulders for support. Keep your knees bent and feet flat as you move up and down or back and forth.

jet jiggy

Facing a jet, kneel on the seat of a hot tub and lean forward so you're on all fours. Have your partner **kneel** between your legs so he can enter you from behind. Once he's firmly inside you, both of you should grab on to the edge of the tub to help balance yourselves and slowly straighten up so the two of you are upright. Continue holding on to the tub for support as he pumps away. With your nether regions directly in the jet stream, you get that all-important clitoral friction, helping you sail closer to the **O zone**.

IN THE SHOWER . . .

hands on the wall

Stand up straight with your hands against the wall and **legs spread slightly**. Your man will enter you from behind. Tip: Be sure to aim your shower head as downward as possible so the water isn't hitting you guys directly in the face. That can be distracting and things will get really wet—not in a good way.

the **seat**

This one always works and you don't risk busting your ass in a slippery bathtub. Have him sit down with his legs stretched out or slightly bent at the knees if he's tall. **Straddle him** and go to town. The water hitting your back lightly will feel extra good.

straight up

Stand up straight with your **back against the wall**, lift one leg up, and wrap it around his lower back. Tip: It will be easier for him to have full control if he presses his hands against the wall you're leaning on.

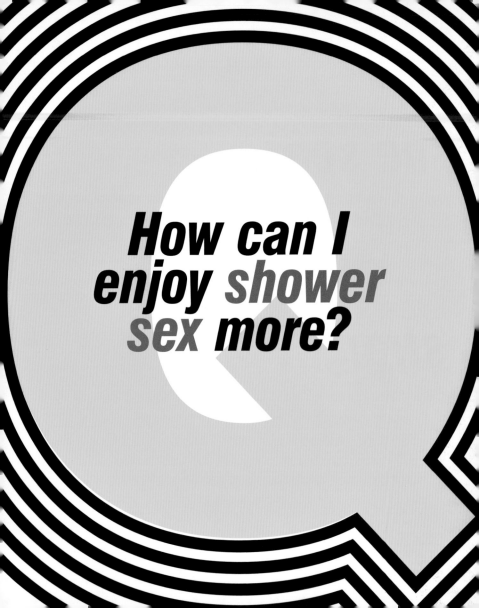

How can I enjoy shower sex more?

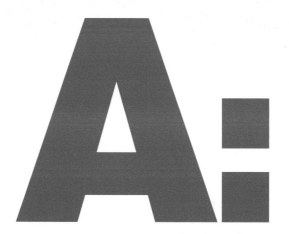

Bring it! Toy time, that is. Megan Andelloux, a clinical sexologist in Pawtucket, Rhode Island, recommends Sex in the Shower, a brand of sex toys with suction handles and footrests that are specifically designed to make getting it on in the tub or shower easier. (If anyone asks what that thing attached to your shower wall is, you can just say it's for shaving.) "I would also suggest some silicone-based lubricant because it stays on in the water," Andelloux says. But hazard warning: Lube does its job so well, it increases your slippage factor if it gets on the shower floor.

WATER WORKS

shower quickie

The shower was practically made for the **quickie**—who wants to linger in there when only one of you can be warm under the water? The ideal position for you is bent over, aiming the shower head at your hot spot while he's doing his thing from behind. No removable shower head? Slick his fingers with shower gel, and have him reach around and give you some digital pleasure.

bathtub sex

In the tub, you loll in his arms while he's behind you. Since water makes you weightless **you can do it** till you prune!

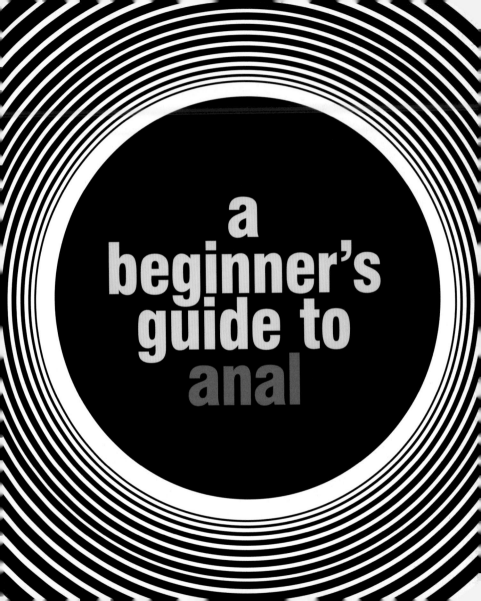

1 **Even if you're monogamous, use a condom.** It prevents bacteria from the bowels spreading anywhere.

----

2 **Choose the right lube.** Between thin water-based lubes (like Astroglide) and thicker ones (KY), go with the thicker ones, because they don't dry out as quickly.

----

3 **Getting the tip in hurts the most.** The head of the penis is the widest part, but once you're past that and up to the shaft, it'll feel a little better.

----

4 **You can lie flat on your stomach, get in doggie style, or do missionary.** But don't do deep penetration until you're ready!

TIP
Anal sex feels best when there's some additional stimulation going on. Vaginal, clitoral, nipple-centric—whichever feels best for you. While some women only need butt play, most women can't come from anal stimulation alone.

anal sex: myth vs. reality

THE MYTH: IT WILL HURT.

THE TRUTH: Anal sex doesn't have to hurt. It's often just done incorrectly. Many women find it incredibly pleasurable, and some even report having orgasms from it. If you and your partner start slow, work your way into insertion with smaller implements like fingers and sex toys, and use plenty of lube, pain will be the last thing on your mind.

THE MYTH: YOU DON'T NEED TO USE CONDOMS WHEN YOU HAVE ANAL SEX.

THE TRUTH: This is a misconception because many people think that because there is no pregnancy risk that you also don't need to use a condom. Wrong, wrong, wrong. Most STDs are transferrable through the anus (chlamydia, gonorrhea, infectious hepatitis, and HIV). Some even more so, because the lining of the anus is much thinner and can be broken more easily if too much dry friction occurs (again, please refer to the importance of lube use).

THE MYTH: IT WILL CAUSE YOU PHYSICAL DAMAGE.

THE TRUTH: Having any sort of sex the "wrong way" could cause damage. Think about it: If you are vaginally dry and don't use additional lube, you can cause microtears in your vagina. The same thing can happen during anal sex. Granted, the vagina does usually create its own lubrication (depending on hormones, etc.) and the anus does not, but that just means real lube (not saliva) needs to be used for a healthy experience.

THE MYTH: YOUR ANUS WILL GET ALL STRETCHED OUT.

THE TRUTH: Just like the myth that the vagina gets irreparably stretched out from childbirth, this is also a misconception. There were rumors in the late seventies of groups of men who engaged in so much anal activity that they actually lost control of bowel movements. Regular, healthy engagement in anal sex will not lead to this outcome. Through regular anal sex, your anus does learn to become more relaxed, but much of that has to do with your ability to relax yourself mentally for the act. And we all know that the vagina accommodates a wide range of penises; the anus can too— with the right introduction.

THE MYTH: IT'S DIRTY (LITERALLY).

THE TRUTH: This is probably one of the biggest misconceptions out there. The anus and the lower part of the rectum actually have very little fecal material in them, which means it tends to not be nearly as dirty as you think. This doesn't mean you should transfer the elements into the vagina by having anal sex and then vaginal sex though, because they are two different environments, and even microscopic fecal elements can cause vaginal infections. Just be sure to wash with antimicrobial soap before vaginal reentry or just end your sexual exploits for that evening with anal sex. Regardless, if you are still concerned, you can always have a bowel movement prior followed by an enema, if you want to be squeaky-clean.

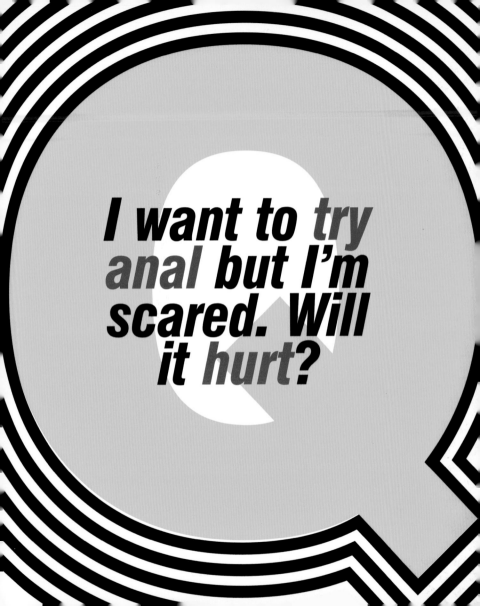

I want to try anal but I'm scared. Will it hurt?

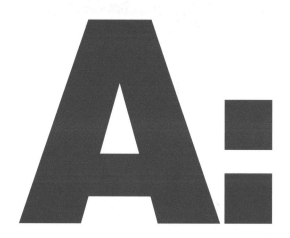

Sex educator Jayne Waxman says before you even *think* about trying it, make sure you have two things: a loving partner who listens, and a good silicone lubricant. "Start with a well-lubricated finger or butt plug before you graduate to a penis," Waxman says. "If your body resists any of those, stop and breathe," she says. "Eventually, when you relax, your rectum will relax with you." Now, as to the second part of your question, yeah, it may hurt a little. It should eventually feel better, even pleasurable. But if it doesn't, don't keep doing it! You may just have a back door that you prefer guests not use.

the
more
the
MERRIER:
threesomes

Because two is nice, but three is company!

WHAT TO KNOW BEFORE

Set clear boundaries about what's okay in the bedroom and out of it—such as whether you will meet your third partner for a date beforehand, and where you'll find them. Will they be male or female, etc.

Agree on a "sacred element" that will remain between just you and your partner, not ever with the third partner.

Set a secret code and agree that if either of you becomes uncomfortable, both partners will end the threesome at once.

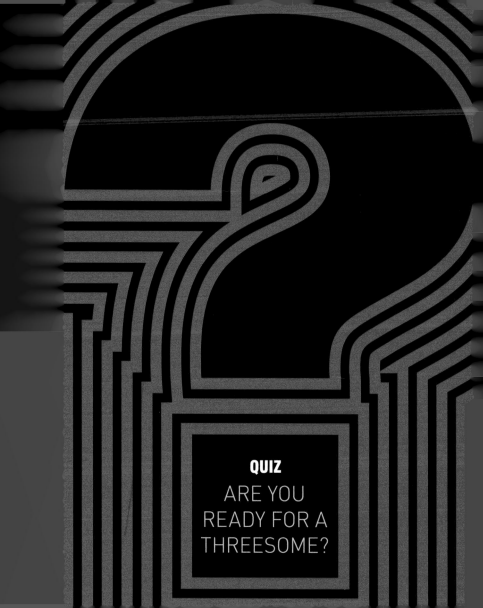

QUIZ

ARE YOU
READY FOR A
THREESOME?

SO YOU AND YOUR GUY are curious about trying a threesome—but how do you know if you're really as cool with it as you think you are?

CHECK ALL THAT APPLY:

___ I've never creeped into my boyfriend's e-mail or text messages.

___ I thought the Marnie-Jessa smooch in *Girls* was kind of hot.

___ I'm pretty adventurous in bed.

___ I'm totally confident about how I look naked.

___ My boyfriend doesn't check out other girls . . . at least not when he's with me.

___ My motto is "I'll try anything once."

___ I am open with my boyfriend about my sexual fantasies and talk about them in detail.

___ I've never stalked my guy's ex on Facebook.

___ I'm down with watching girl-on-girl porn sometimes.

___ The idea of pleasuring two guys at once is a turn-on.

___ When it comes to men, my motto is "one is fun, but two is twice as nice!"

IF YOU DON'T AGREE WITH AT LEAST SEVEN OF THESE STATEMENTS, you may regret adding another girl (or guy) to the mix. No matter how comfortable you are with sex, having a threesome with your boyfriend and someone else can bring up all kinds of issues afterward—especially jealousy. Unless you're totally confident in yourself, 100 percent secure in your relationship, sexually curious, a little bit kinky, and somewhat attracted to chicks, you might think twice before giving the green light to a three-way.

My boyfriend and I are dying to have a **threesome** with another girl. Where do we even *begin*?

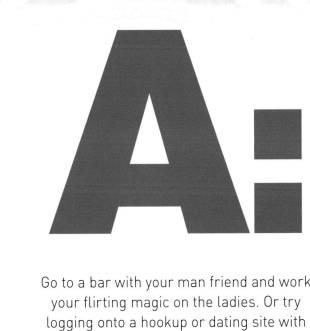

Go to a bar with your man friend and work your flirting magic on the ladies. Or try logging onto a hookup or dating site with threesome categories. Single ladies are looking for couples to get down with on PolyMatchmaker and OkCupid. Whether you pick her up online or in person, discuss the rules and what's on the sexual menu before you get naked. And use condoms!

SEX HOLIDAYS

to celebrate all year long

January
8

NATIONAL BUBBLE BATH DAY

Even though it was probably created with bath oils and Enya in mind, use this (real) holiday as an excuse to hop into the tub—armed with waterproof lube, of course—and get down and dirty.

February
15

SINGLES AWARENESS DAY

Who needs Tinder when you have . . . you? Shamelessly make yourself dinner, tell yourself you're hotter than Kate Upton, unsheath your favorite vibe, and revel in solo sex.

March
(falls on a Sunday in early or mid March)

DAYLIGHT SAVINGS

Pissed about losing an hour's sleep? Make it up to yourself with a bonus hour of sex. Why not use that extra daylight for a sunny girl-on-top session? Pre-work orgasms make you spring forward a lot faster than a latte.

April
22

EARTH DAY

Bees do it, birds do it . . . you know where we're going with this, yes? Honor Mother Nature by getting it on in the great outdoors—under a tree, in the ocean, on a mountain—the sky's the limit. What? It's only natural.

May
5

CINCO DE MAYO

We'll spare you the crude taco joke, but for this celebration of all things Mexican, literally take your fiesta south of the border: Challenge yourselves to drive each other wild with only your mouths.

June
14

FLAG DAY

Celebrate the adoption of the American stars and stripes by pledging allegiance to your own freak flag. Today, act out the secret kinky fantasy you've been hiding: Tie him up, ask for a spanking, eat chocolate cake in bed. . . . It's the patriotic thing to do.

VALENTINE'S DAY SEX is so obvious, as are anniversary BJs. Here's a year's worth of new reasons to pop the champers and get it on.

July
14 BASTILLE DAY

In honor of the French Revolution, storm *his* Bastille. Try a textured French tickler–style condom, and bust out dirty talk galore—after all, French is the language of love.

August
25 KISS AND MAKE UP DAY

Spark a playful *Homeland* vs. *Breaking Bad* debate with your guy. When you start feeling as heated as your convo, break the tension by hiking up your dress and having impromptu sex right on the spot.

September
(starts every year on a Saturday in mid September)

OKTOBERFEST

No need to fly to Germany—a frisky fräulein like you can make a rowdy party right at home. Slip on your sexiest thigh-highs, mount your man's . . . bratwurst, and get as loud as a bustling beer garden.

October
22 COLUMBUS DAY

Let Columbus inspire a little sexploration: Tie your man's hands behind his back, and allow him to venture anywhere on your body . . . but only with his mouth. If you happen to be on a boat, all the better. Whole new world, indeed.

November
15 AMERICA RECYCLES DAY

Reduce, reuse . . . relive your best sex ever. Wax nostalgic over the hottest nights you've had—remember the Great Blended Orgasm of '09?—and incorporate them into tonight's routine.

December
26 BOXING DAY

This British holiday is all about gift boxes stuffed with goodies. This can mean only one thing: DIY sex box! Fill a leftover Christmas box with a paddle, some warming lube, and a glow-in-the-dark condom—and invite him to celebrate the final days of the holiday season.

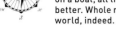

333

NOW, GO

AND CO

SEX GO

VALENTINE'S DAY SEX is so obvious, as are anniversary BJs. Here's a year's worth of new reasons to pop the champers and get it on.

July
14

BASTILLE DAY

In honor of the French Revolution, storm *his* Bastille. Try a textured French tickler–style condom, and bust out dirty talk galore—after all, French is the language of love.

August
25

KISS AND MAKE UP DAY

Spark a playful *Homeland* vs. *Breaking Bad* debate with your guy. When you start feeling as heated as your convo, break the tension by hiking up your dress and having impromptu sex right on the spot.

September
(starts every year on a Saturday in mid September)

OKTOBERFEST

No need to fly to Germany—a frisky fräulein like you can make a rowdy party right at home. Slip on your sexiest thigh-highs, mount your man's . . . bratwurst, and get as loud as a bustling beer garden.

October
22

COLUMBUS DAY

Let Columbus inspire a little sexploration: Tie your man's hands behind his back, and allow him to venture anywhere on your body . . . but only with his mouth. If you happen to be on a boat, all the better. Whole new world, indeed.

November
15

AMERICA RECYCLES DAY

Reduce, reuse . . . relive your best sex ever. Wax nostalgic over the hottest nights you've had—remember the Great Blended Orgasm of '09?—and incorporate them into tonight's routine.

December
26

BOXING DAY

This British holiday is all about gift boxes stuffed with goodies. This can mean only one thing: DIY sex box! Fill a leftover Christmas box with a paddle, some warming lube, and a glow-in-the-dark condom—and invite him to celebrate the final days of the holiday season.

NOW, GO
AND CO
SEX GO

O FORTH

NQUER,

DDESS!

HEARST BOOKS
New York

An Imprint of Sterling Publishing
1166 Avenue of the Americas
New York, NY 10036

Cosmopolitan is a registered trademark of Hearst Communications, Inc.

ISBN 978-1-61837-193-5

Cover Design: Phil Buchanan
Credits:
Cover photo: © Blossom Berkofsky
Sex position illustrations by Timothy Hunt

© Blossom Berkofsky: 8; © Emmet Malström: 66; © Tamara Schlesinger: 234; Studio D: Ben Goldstein: 239,
241, 243; Getty Images: © ballyscanlon: 332 top left; © Lauren Burke: 333 bottom left; © C Squared Studios:
333 top left; © Comstock Images: 333 top right; © Creative Crop: 332 right; © Rebecca Ellis: 332 center;
© Majchrzak Morel: 332 bottom left; © Pingebat: 333 bottom left

Distributed in Canada by Sterling Publishing
c/o Canadian Manda Group, 664 Annette Street
Toronto, Ontario, Canada M6S 2C8
Distributed in the United Kingdom by GMC Distribution Services
Castle Place, 166 High Street, Lewes, East Sussex, England BN7 1XU
Distributed in Australia by Capricorn Link (Australia) Pty. Ltd.
P.O. Box 704, Windsor, NSW 2756, Australia

For information about custom editions, special sales, and premium and
corporate purchases, please contact Sterling Special Sales at 800-805-5489
or specialsales@sterlingpublishing.com

Manufactured in China

2 4 6 8 10 9 7 5 3 1

www.sterlingpublishing.com